THE
EVERYTHING®
GUIDE TO
THE MIND DIET

Dear Reader,

My journey to health and wellness did not happen overnight. Like many of us I was overweight, letting my health deteriorate gradually as I prioritized other parts of my life. Unlike most of us though, as a physician I thought I had the tools and knowledge to avoid such health pitfalls. Watching my mind and body decline, I recognized that by not taking adequate care of myself, I was not taking adequate care of those around me.

After turning my own health around, I became passionate about doing the same for others. I also learned that for a change in lifestyle to be sustainable, it has to be simple.

Fortunately, new research is revealing that by simply eating certain foods and exercising, not only can we better preserve our bodies, but we can sustain our minds through old age as well. Preventing Alzheimer's, dementia, and other forms of mental decline may be as simple as making good choices now. And you can get started today.

The Everything® Guide to the MIND Diet will help guide you in making the right choices to take control of your mental and physical health, starting now and for the rest of your life.

Yours in health,

Murdoc Khaleghi, MD

Welcome to the EVERYTHING® Series!

These handy, accessible books give you all you need to tackle a difficult project, gain a new hobby, comprehend a fascinating topic, prepare for an exam, or even brush up on something you learned back in school but have since forgotten.

You can choose to read an Everything® book from cover to cover or just pick out the information you want from our four useful boxes: e-questions, e-facts, e-alerts, and e-ssentials.

We give you everything you need to know on the subject, but throw in a lot of fun stuff along the way, too.

We now have more than 400 Everything® books in print, spanning such wide-ranging categories as weddings, pregnancy, cooking, music instruction, foreign language, crafts, pets, New Age, and so much more. When you're done reading them all, you can finally say you know Everything®!

QUESTION

Answers to
common questions

FACT

Important snippets
of information

ALERT

Urgent
warnings

ESSENTIAL

Quick
handy tips

PUBLISHER Karen Cooper

MANAGING EDITOR Lisa Laing

COPY CHIEF Casey Ebert

ASSISTANT PRODUCTION EDITOR Jo-Anne Duhamel

ACQUISITIONS EDITOR Hillary Thompson

DEVELOPMENT EDITOR Katie Corcoran Lytle

EVERYTHING® SERIES COVER DESIGNER Erin Alexander

Visit the entire Everything® series at www.everything.com

THE
EVERYTHING®
GUIDE TO
THE MIND DIET

Optimize brain health and prevent disease
with nutrient-dense foods

Christy Ellingsworth and Murdoc Khaleghi, MD

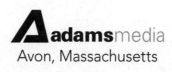

adamsmedia
Avon, Massachusetts

Dedicated to Laura, Andy, Alyssa, and PJ. Thanks for keeping my mind sharp!

An Everything® Series Book.
Everything® and everything.com® are registered trademarks of F+W Media, Inc.

Published by
Adams Media, a division of F+W Media, Inc.
57 Littlefield Street, Avon, MA 02322. U.S.A.
www.adamsmedia.com

Contains material adapted from *The Everything® Low-Salt Cookbook* by Pamela Rice Hahn, copyright © 2004 by F+W Media, Inc., ISBN 10: 1-59337-044-X, ISBN 13: 978-1-59337-044-2; *The Everything® DASH Diet Cookbook* by Christy Ellingsworth and Murdoc Khaleghi, MD, copyright © 2012 by F+W Media, Inc., ISBN 10: 1-4405-4353-4, ISBN 13: 978-1-4405-4353-1; and *The DASH Diet 30-Minute Cookbook* by Christy Ellingsworth, copyright © 2015 by F+W Media, Inc., ISBN 10: 1-4405-9072-9, ISBN 13: 978-1-4405-9072-6.

ISBN 10: 1-4405-9799-5
ISBN 13: 978-1-4405-9799-2
eISBN 10: 1-4405-9800-2
eISBN 13: 978-1-4405-9800-5

Printed in the United States of America.

10 9 8 7 6 5 4 3 2 1

Library of Congress Cataloging-in-Publication Data

Ellingsworth, Christy, author. | Khaleghi, Murdoc, author.
The everything guide to the MIND diet / Christy Ellingsworth and Murdoc Khaleghi, MD.
Avon, Massachusetts: Adams Media, 2016.
Series: An everything series book.
Includes bibliographical references and index.
Identifiers: LCCN 2016021759 (print) | LCCN 2016023017 (ebook) | ISBN 9781440597992 (pb) | ISBN 1440597995 (pb) | ISBN 9781440598005 (ebook) | ISBN 1440598002 (ebook)
LCSH: Brain--Diseases--Prevention--Popular works. | Brain--Diseases--Nutritional aspects. | Cooking. | BISAC: HEALTH & FITNESS / Diets. | COOKING / Health & Healing / Low Fat.
LCC RC386.2 .E45 2016 (print) | LCC RC386.2 (ebook) | DDC 616.8/04654--dc23
LC record available at https://lccn.loc.gov/2016021759

Cover image © StockFood/Scherer, Jim.
Nutritional statistics by Melinda Boyd, MPH, MHR, RD.

*This book is available at quantity discounts for bulk purchases.
For information, please call 1-800-289-0963.*

Contents

Introduction

BRAIN HEALTH HAS BEEN receiving more attention in society as of late, and for good reason. As we become older, our cognition—our ability to think—declines. This is particularly worrisome and challenging as the size of the U.S. population entering their golden years is quickly growing. This decline can come in various forms, from minor forgetfulness and getting slower at answering *Jeopardy!* questions to neurodegenerative disorders such as Alzheimer's disease (AD), where in its severest form a person may have no memory of the past or awareness of the current situation. Many physicians and researchers suggest that the increasing prevalence of AD is not only due to an aging population but changes in our diet over the past century. Because of the severe effects of dementia and other forms of mental decline, more people are starting to care about how their diet affects the mind as well as the body.

The MIND diet—short for Mediterranean-DASH Intervention for Neurodegenerative Delay—attempts to reverse the ongoing trend of mental decline and prevent disease while helping you lose weight and boosting energy. By adopting features of two of the most popular diets that have been studied and touted for their beneficial health effects—the Mediterranean and DASH (Dietary Approaches to Stop Hypertension) diets—the MIND diet focuses on adopting foods that can protect the brain and steers you away from foods that are damaging to your body and brain health.

Perhaps most importantly, research is showing that the MIND diet may prevent the onset of Alzheimer's. In fact, no diet has demonstrated as much potential for the prevention of AD as the MIND diet. One study of the MIND diet through the Rush University Medical Center specifically showed a reduction in risk of Alzheimer's by more than 50 percent! In addition, *U.S. News & World Report* has named the MIND diet one of the easiest diets to follow. If you are hoping to protect your brain with a stress-free plan, the MIND diet is an ideal combination of effectiveness and ease to make it the right diet for you!

The simplicity of the MIND diet is that it allows many types of foods you can eat while only discouraging a few types. Specifically, foods promoted by the MIND diet include vegetables—especially the green leafy kind—as well as nuts, berries, beans, whole grains, fish, poultry, olive oil, and even wine. Foods discouraged include red meat, butter and margarine, cheese, pastries and sweets, and fried or processed fast food.

Rather than having to be overly restrictive, you merely have to direct yourself away from harmful foods and toward more healthful choices. And with the 200 delicious recipes in this book, you'll have plenty of healthy meals and snacks to choose from.

This book is a comprehensive yet easy-to-understand guide on the importance of protecting your brain. By making simple choices now, you can support your brain health, and overall health, now and into the future.

CHAPTER 1

What Is the MIND Diet?

In February 2015, a study was published in the medical journal *Alzheimer's & Dementia* that blew everyone's minds. According to the researchers, older adults who followed a specific diet, called the Mediterranean-DASH Intervention for Neurodegenerative Delay diet, or the MIND diet, were able to reduce their risk of developing Alzheimer's disease—and rather significantly. In fact, the study participants who followed the diet to the letter saw reductions in Alzheimer's disease risk of up to 53 percent. The MIND diet is a combination of two diets that have been both successful and wildly popular for some time: the Mediterranean diet and the DASH (Dietary Approaches to Stop Hypertension) diet.

In this chapter you'll learn how and why the MIND diet was developed and the foods that are included and excluded. You'll also learn about the two diets from which the MIND diet was developed.

The Foods That Affect Brain Health

Like the Mediterranean and DASH diets, the MIND diet emphasizes the consumption of plant-based foods and healthy fats while limiting the consumption of animal products and foods that are high in saturated fat. In addition to the healthy fats, the stars of the diet are berries and green leafy vegetables.

The MIND diet is built around fifteen dietary components—ten of these components are brain-healthy foods that make up the bulk of the diet, and the other five are foods that are considered unhealthy and are restricted while following the diet.

TEN BRAIN-HEALTHY FOODS TO INCLUDE

- Beans
- Blueberries
- Fish
- Green leafy vegetables (e.g. spinach, kale, lettuce, and arugula)
- Nuts
- Olive oil
- Other vegetables (e.g. sweet potatoes, asparagus, and cauliflower)
- Poultry
- Whole grains
- Red wine

FIVE BRAIN-UNHEALTHY FOODS TO AVOID

- Butter and margarine
- Cheese
- Fried foods
- Pastries and desserts
- Red meat

According to research, the more closely the diet is followed, the greater the positive impact on your brain health.

Research Findings and Diet Success

Dr. Martha Clare Morris, a nutritional epidemiologist at Rush University Medical Center, developed the MIND diet. The 2015 study, which was funded by the National Institute on Aging, followed the food intake of 923 Chicago-area senior citizens over a period of four and a half years. After this time, researchers found that 144 of the study participants developed Alzheimer's disease while the remaining study participants did not. The researchers concluded that the longer and more closely participants followed the diet, the less risk they had of developing Alzheimer's disease and other cognitive impairment.

Study participants who followed the MIND diet "moderately well" showed a 35 percent reduction in risk of developing Alzheimer's disease, while those who strictly adhered to the program experienced a 53 percent reduction in Alzheimer's risk.

ESSENTIAL

More than 5 million Americans are living with Alzheimer's disease or another form of dementia. Alzheimer's disease is currently the sixth-leading cause of death in the United States. The disease kills more people than prostate cancer and breast cancer combined.

Alzheimer's Disease and Dementia

Before we dive deeper into how food plays a role in your memory and the health of your brain in general, let's take a quick look at what Alzheimer's disease and dementia are—and the known risk factors for developing them.

Dementia is not a specific disease; it's a general term that describes a decline in memory, thinking skills, and cognition that is severe enough to interfere with a person's ability to perform normal, everyday activities. Alzheimer's disease, which is the most common form of dementia, accounts for 60–80 percent of cases. While symptoms of dementia and Alzheimer's disease can vary from person to person, some of the most common include:

- Impaired memory
- Reduced communication and language skills
- Inability to focus
- Decrease in reasoning and judgment
- Impaired visual perception

Most forms of dementia are progressive, which means the symptoms start out gradual and then get worse as time goes on.

The Workings of Your Brain

Your brain contains 100 billion nerve cells, called neurons. Each one of these neurons connects with many others to form communication networks all over the brain and the rest of your body. Some of these neurons are involved in thinking, learning, and remembering past events and new information, while others help you move or see or smell. Your brain is the control center of your body, and in order for it to work properly there must be flawless communication between all of these neural networks.

Researchers have identified some risk factors that increase the likelihood of developing Alzheimer's disease and other neurodegenerative disorders, but there are still a lot of questions that remain unanswered. One thing that researchers do agree on, however, is that somewhere, somehow, neurons become damaged and are unable to do their job. As the damage spreads, more cells become affected and some begin to die off. It's the death of these nerve cells that causes the symptoms that are characteristic of Alzheimer's disease.

Alzheimer's Disease Symptoms

The most common initial symptom of Alzheimer's disease is difficulty remembering newly learned information. Like other forms of dementia, as Alzheimer's advances, the symptoms gradually become worse. Someone with Alzheimer's disease may experience disorientation; mood and behavior changes; unfounded suspicions about family members and friends; difficulty speaking, swallowing, and walking; and worsening memory loss. Often, it's not the person directly affected by Alzheimer's disease that first notices there's an issue but close family members or friends.

Risk Factors

The greatest known risk factor for developing dementia and Alzheimer's disease is advancing age. One out of nine people aged sixty-five or older have Alzheimer's; one out of three aged eighty-five or older are affected. Another known risk factor for Alzheimer's is genetics. If you have a family member who has been affected by Alzheimer's, you are more likely to become affected as well. However, when discussing genes, it is important to note that there are two different types: risk genes and deterministic genes.

Risk genes increase the likelihood of developing a disease, but don't guarantee that you'll actually get that disease. Researchers have identified several different risk genes that may be involved in the development of Alzheimer's disease. Deterministic genes directly cause a disease. This means that anyone who inherits a deterministic gene is guaranteed to be affected by the associated disease or disorder. Although researchers have identified deterministic genes to be the cause of some cases of Alzheimer's, they are implicated in a very small percentage—or only a few hundred families worldwide—and account for fewer than 5 percent of cases.

A gene is a compound that tells your body how to make a protein. Proteins control all cellular functions, so defects in a gene can cause the improper creation of a protein. As a result, that protein prevents certain cells from functioning the way they're supposed to. Genes are made of DNA and are carried on the chromosomes in a cell's nucleus. Most genes are present in pairs, since you get one chromosome from each parent.

Most experts agree that the majority of Alzheimer's cases develop as a result of complex interactions between a variety of factors, including risk genes, age, and lifestyle. While you can't change your heredity or your family history, you can change your lifestyle, which includes the food you're eating. If you eat in a way that prohibits certain genes from expressing themselves, you may be able to prevent diseases like Alzheimer's or even reduce the severity of symptoms once they develop.

Memory, Cognition, and Food

For years, researchers have been working to uncover some answers about what you can do to prevent Alzheimer's disease and other memory problems and even treat them once they develop. Dr. Scott Small, the director of the Alzheimer's Disease Research Center at Columbia University, states that while memory may decline with age, it may not be inevitable. He goes on to suggest that as researchers understand the vital role that food and nutrients play in brain function and health, more natural approaches for treatment, like diet and supplementation, can be developed. That's where the MIND diet comes into play.

The nutrients in food are synergistic, meaning that they work together to provide you with various health benefits. You need all the recommended nutrients, in different amounts, to stay healthy. That being said, researchers have isolated a few specific nutrients as some of the primary reasons for the positive results in the aforementioned studies.

Vitamin E

All of the tissues in your body contain lipids (fats and other fatty compounds) as part of the cell membranes, but your brain is particularly rich in these substances. Unfortunately, lipids are extremely susceptible to oxidative damage, the breakdown in DNA structure due to exposure to free radicals—unstable and highly reactive compounds that damage cells. Add to this the fact that your brain uses up a lot more oxygen in relation to its size than other parts of your body and you have a double whammy for the potential for oxidative stress. In simple terms, oxidative stress is what happens when the amount of free radicals (unstable substances that cause damage to your cells) in your body becomes too high to be neutralized by the antioxidants in your body. Antioxidants, which you can get from the foods you eat, counteract free radicals, preventing them from causing any harm to your cells. Enter vitamin E.

FACT

Vitamin E is not a single compound but rather a group of eight different compounds that are closely related. Four of these substances are called tocopherols and four are called tocotrienols. The most biologically active of the vitamin E compounds is called alpha-tocopherol.

Vitamins come in two forms: fat-soluble and water-soluble. Vitamin E is fat-soluble, which means that it dissolves in fat and is carried through the body in globules of fat, called chylomicrons. These chylomicrons travel through your lymphatic system before entering the small intestine and finally reaching the bloodstream. From there, vitamin E is stored in fatty tissues, like your brain.

In addition to its classification as a fat-soluble vitamin, vitamin E is also a powerful antioxidant. When it reaches your brain, it helps neutralize free radicals, rendering them harmless. This process protects your brain from cognitive decline and the development of degenerative diseases, like Alzheimer's.

The association between brain health and vitamin E extends beyond free radicals and antioxidant power, though. An Oregon State University study, published in the *Journal of Lipid Research*, examined zebrafish that were deficient in vitamin E. Researchers discovered that these zebrafish had 30 percent lower levels of DHA-PC, a component of the cellular membranes of the neurons in the brain. Research from other studies suggests that low levels of DHA-PC in humans are associated with an increased risk of developing Alzheimer's disease because when DHA-PC is low, neurons, which are responsible for a number of functions including memory, cannot perform correctly. Although the study was an animal study, its implications for human health are significant since DHA-PC is a vital component in human neuron as well.

FACT

In the United States, it's estimated that 96 percent of adult women and 90 percent of adult men do not get enough vitamin E in their diet. That means that a large majority of adults may be walking around vitamin E–deficient without even realizing it.

Omega-3 Fatty Acids

Omega-3 fatty acids are a form of polyunsaturated fat that are considered essential. When a nutrient is essential, it means that the body cannot make it, so you must obtain it from food. The connection between omega-3 fatty acids and heart health has been widely documented, but what's discussed less frequently is their extremely important role in brain health. Omega-3 fatty acids account for approximately 8 percent of the brain's weight. Both the omega-3 fatty acids docosahexaenoic acid (DHA) and eicosapentaenoic acid (EPA) play various roles in the function and structure of the brain's neurons.

DHA and EPA protect the brain from oxidative damage, chronic inflammation, and other substances that may cause harm. Studies have shown that this balance of fatty acids in the brain has a major impact on whether a particular neuron will be protected from inflammation or injury, or whether it will become damaged.

Omega-3 fatty acids accumulate in the brain during fetal development, but tend to decline with age if the diet lacks the nutrients to compensate for this natural loss. Several studies demonstrate that levels of DHA tend to be lower in the brains and blood plasma of Alzheimer's patients than in those of elderly individuals without cognitive impairment. Other studies show that people with dementia who were treated with fish oil capsules that offered 1,400 milligrams of DHA per day showed marked improvement in brain function. This has led scientists to suggest that the cognitive decline associated with Alzheimer's disease and other brain-related chronic diseases is at least in part connected to this natural deterioration of omega-3 fatty acids in the brain's cell membranes.

ESSENTIAL

Omega-3 fatty acids are classified as essential nutrients. Essential nutrients are those that your body cannot make but that you need to stay healthy. Because your body cannot make essential nutrients, you need to get them through your diet.

As a society, we tend to accept a faltering memory as a normal part of advancing age, but it seems that a diet rich in omega-3 fatty acids can help ensure that this, along with dementia and Alzheimer's, isn't an accepted part of the aging process.

Micronutrients

In addition to vitamin E and omega-3 fatty acids, the brain needs a constant supply of various micronutrients for proper energy metabolism of neurons—the cells that transmit nerve impulses—and glial cells, which insulate and support neurons. The brain is also a highly metabolically active tissue, meaning it constantly uses energy and must have access to a steady supply of glucose (from the food you eat) to meet its energy needs.

In order for glucose to be utilized by the brain, it requires the presence of certain micronutrients. These micronutrients—specifically the B vitamins thiamin, riboflavin, niacin, and pantothenic acid, as well as lipoic acid and the minerals magnesium, iron, and manganese—act as cofactors, which are substances that allow chemical reactions to take place. Without proper amounts of these micronutrients, the brain cannot obtain the energy it needs to function properly. The MIND diet optimizes micronutrient intake by encouraging the consumption of nutrient-dense foods like vegetables, berries, nuts, seeds, and oils, and it discourages the consumption of nutrient-poor filler foods like sweets and fried foods. These nutrient-dense foods also give your brain access to the glucose it needs.

The DASH Diet

The National Heart, Lung, and Blood Institute promotes the DASH (Dietary Approaches to Stop Hypertension) diet as a way for people with hypertension to help control their blood pressure. In addition to encouraging those following the dietary program to reduce their intake of sodium, the DASH diet promotes an increased consumption of magnesium, calcium, and potassium—three minerals that play a role in maintaining a healthy blood pressure. The DASH diet also emphasizes consumption of a large amount of foods that are rich in antioxidants, which not only ward off the development of heart problems but help prevent chronic degenerative diseases like Alzheimer's, too.

Because research shows that the DASH diet has been effective at preventing chronic diseases, the creators of the MIND diet took some components of the DASH diet when creating the new diet plan. Unlike the DASH diet, however, the MIND diet doesn't include a restriction on salt or sodium, since the main focus is on brain health, rather than heart health.

Diet Components

The DASH diet centers around fruits, vegetables, low-fat dairy products, and whole grains. It also encourages the consumption of legumes, poultry, and fish and allows small amounts of red meat, fats, and sweets. It is low in sodium, saturated fat, total fat, and cholesterol.

The diet is broken down as follows (each recommendation is per day unless otherwise indicated):

- Six to eight servings of grains
- Four or five servings of vegetables
- Four or five servings of fruits
- Two or three servings of low-fat dairy
- Four or five servings of nuts, seeds, and legumes
- Two or three servings of fats and oils
- Up to six servings of fish, poultry, or lean meats
- Up to five servings of sweets per week (e.g. chocolate, cookies, and ice cream)
- No more than two alcoholic beverages per day for men and no more than one per day for women

Although sweets are not expressly forbidden on the MIND diet, it's best to limit them as much as possible. The MIND diet allows for up to five servings per week, but keep your intake as low as you can. Sugar provides nothing but empty calories and foods that are high in sugar are typically low in the micronutrients that contribute to your brain health.

How Effective Is the DASH Diet?

The DASH diet is so effective that it has been the primary diet recommended for patients with high blood pressure and/or heart disease since 1997. The DASH diet can significantly lower blood pressure in those with high blood pressure, which in turn, also lowers the risk of developing heart disease.

Research published in the medical journal *Hypertension* found that patients with prehypertension, or blood pressure that was slightly elevated but not enough to be classified as true high blood pressure, experienced an average drop of 6 mm Hg in systolic blood pressure (or the top number of a blood pressure reading) and 3 mm Hg in diastolic blood pressure (or the bottom number of a blood pressure reading) when following the DASH diet. Patients who were diagnosed with hypertension, or high blood pressure, experienced reductions of 11 mm Hg in systolic blood pressure and 6 mm Hg in diastolic blood pressure, on average. So what does this mean? It means that people who follow the DASH diet experience a significant reduction in their blood pressure, even without the use of medications. These benefits, along with the added benefit of brain health, are carried over when the DASH diet's recommendations are combined with those of the Mediterranean diet to create the MIND diet.

The Mediterranean Diet

Like the DASH diet, the Mediterranean diet was originally developed with heart health in mind. As the name implies, the Mediterranean diet was modeled after the eating habits and traditional foods people ate in Mediterranean countries like Italy and Greece in the 1960s. After studying the Mediterranean people, researchers concluded that they were remarkably healthier than Americans and that they had much lower rates of chronic diseases like heart disease and Type 2 diabetes.

The benefits didn't end there, though. Researchers also found that the Mediterranean people had lower incidences of neurodegenerative diseases, like Alzheimer's disease. The creators of the MIND diet recognized this significance, and as a result, took several components of the Mediterranean diet when developing the MIND diet.

Diet Components

Unlike the DASH diet, which tends to be more of a therapeutic diet, the Mediterranean diet doesn't have any specific guidelines for how many servings of each type of food you are required to eat each day. Instead, the Mediterranean diet plan is based on its own food pyramid.

At the bottom of the pyramid are the foods that make up the bulk of the diet. These foods, which should be eaten daily, include fruits, vegetables, nuts, seeds, legumes, potatoes, whole grains, and extra-virgin olive oil. Fish and seafood are the next step on the pyramid, and it's recommended to consume these foods at least twice per week. As you move up the pyramid, you get to poultry, eggs, cheese, and yogurt, which should only be eaten in moderation (only two times per week at most). At the top of the pyramid lies red meat and sweets (added sugar), which should be eaten rarely (no more than once a month), if at all.

The Mediterranean diet is unique because it emphasizes that you should make an effort to not only enjoy your meals but to also eat with others. The pyramid also stresses daily physical activity. In fact, exercise and enjoying your meals with others provides the foundation (or the largest section) of the pyramid.

How Effective Is It?

Although the Mediterranean diet was designed to improve heart health, researchers found that following the diet also led to reduced incidences of cancer, Parkinson's disease, and Alzheimer's disease. This prompted researchers, like Martha Morris, the developer of the MIND diet, to dig further into what components of the diet were responsible for these improvements in brain health and whether the power of those dietary components could be harnessed and turned into a "brain-healthy" diet. The researchers decided that the best way to improve brain health and prevent Alzheimer's disease was to combine specific components of the two diets. They took the emphasis on healthy fat from the Mediterranean diet while the recommendation for a high intake of antioxidants came from both diet plans.

Developing the MIND Diet

As you can see, there is growing evidence that links your heart health to your brain health. Every time your heart beats, it pumps approximately 20–25 percent of the blood in your body to your head, where the cells in your brain use up 20 percent of the nutrients and oxygen that your blood carries. Because of this intricate connection between your vascular system and your brain, it makes sense that the risk of developing Alzheimer's disease increases with the presence of conditions like high blood pressure, stroke, heart disease, high cholesterol, and diabetes—which all affect your heart and/or your vascular system.

When developing the MIND diet, Martha Morris took the info that she learned from her study results and combined it with the success of the DASH diet and the Mediterranean diet to create an easy-to-follow diet plan that helps to improve brain function. Similar to both the DASH diet and the Mediterranean diet, the MIND diet emphasizes a plant-based diet plan.

Unlike the other two diets, though, the MIND diet specifically encourages the consumption of green leafy vegetables and berries—two powerful foods for brain health.

Morris's plan was very successful. In 2016, the MIND diet was ranked number 1 in the *U.S. News & World Report*'s "Easiest Diet to Follow" category and number 2 in the "Best Diet Overall" category. So now that you know how the MIND diet was created, let's take a closer look at what you should be eating—and why you should be eating it—when you're following the plan.

CHAPTER 2

What to Eat and Why

When Dr. Morris developed the MIND diet, she had two major goals in mind. The first was to create a diet plan that could improve brain health and cut the risk of developing devastating neurodegenerative disorders like Alzheimer's disease significantly. The second was to ensure that the diet was easy to follow, so that people would actually stick to the program and see the results they were after. Unlike the Mediterranean and DASH diets, the MIND diet doesn't have strict daily recommendations for each group or for specific minerals, like sodium. Instead, the MIND diet gives general recommendations, either daily or weekly, with a few guidelines that should be followed every day. In this chapter, you'll learn what you should (and shouldn't) be eating on the MIND diet and why.

Healthy Food Categories

The two main underlying factors that lead to neurodegenerative diseases are inflammation and oxidative stress—which happens when the production of free radicals, which come from a poor diet, excess stress, and toxins (like pollution or cigarette smoke) in the body is greater than your body's ability to neutralize those free radicals through antioxidants. In order to prevent neurodegenerative diseases from developing, you have to eliminate chronic inflammation and combat oxidative stress. There are several ways to do that. One, of course, is to alter your eating habits. This is the main principle of the MIND diet.

The MIND diet is built around fifteen major food categories—ten of these categories are healthy foods that provide the foundation of the diet, and the other five categories are foods that should be avoided or limited while following the plan. The ten "brain-healthy foods" provide different nutrients that help boost cognitive function and improve memory and learning skills; the five "brain-unhealthy foods" are foods that contribute to cognitive decline and may even play a role in the development of Alzheimer's disease and other forms of dementia.

The ten healthy categories are made up of the following foods. In addition to these staple foods, you can also enjoy low-fat yogurt, other legumes like lentils, and other healthy fats like avocado, coconut, and olives as part of your plan. These foods should not take the place of the daily staples, but they are okay to include with your meals.

- Green leafy vegetables—at least six servings per week
- Other vegetables—at least one per day
- Nuts—at least five servings per week
- Blueberries—two or more servings per week
- Whole grains—three or more servings per day
- Beans—at least three servings per week
- Fish—at least one serving per week
- Poultry—at least two servings per week
- Olive oil—consume daily (use as your main cooking oil)
- Red wine—one glass (4–5 ounces) per day

Let's take a closer look at these brain-healthy foods . . .

Green Leafy Vegetables

Green leafy vegetables are one of the main focuses of the MIND diet—and for good reason. They are loaded with nutrients that perform a wide range of functions to keep you healthy, but there are some specific vitamins that give the greens their brain-boosting power.

In a study led by Morris, researchers tracked the diets and cognitive abilities of 923 older adults (with an average age of eighty-one) for a period of four and a half years. The researchers witnessed a rapid decrease in the rate of cognitive decline in the study participants who consumed the largest amount of leafy green vegetables, which are rich in vitamin K. The study participants who ate one or two servings of leafy greens per day had cognitive abilities equivalent to a person eleven years younger when compared to participants who consumed no leafy greens. Researchers believe that in addition to folate, lutein, and beta carotene, vitamin K is largely responsible for this effect.

FACT

At birth, your brain was almost the same size as an adult brain and contained almost all of the brain cells you'll have your whole life. The brain officially stops growing at the age of eighteen so the actual size of it remains the same no matter how old you get.

As a result of these significant findings, Morris made leafy green vegetables the foundation of the MIND diet to ensure that those following the plan would be taking in plenty of vitamin K.

Other Vegetables

Although leafy greens are one of the vegetable powerhouses of the MIND diet program, other vegetables are included in the diet as well. Brightly colored vegetables, like carrots and squash, and cruciferous vegetables, like broccoli and cauliflower, are also loaded with beta carotene and antioxidants that protect the brain from damage from free radicals and help ward off inflammation, which can put stress on the brain and reduce both short-term and long-term memory.

Nuts

It might be a coincidence that walnuts look like tiny brains in a shell—or maybe it's Mother Nature providing hints of their brain-boosting power. Walnuts are high in alpha-linolenic acid—a plant-based omega-3 fatty acid that is known to ward off Alzheimer's disease. They are also extremely high in antioxidants, which protect against inflammation and cell damage, and magnesium, which can help the heart cope under the pressure of stressful times.

In a study performed at the New York State Institute for Basic Research in Developmental Disabilities, researchers found that Alzheimer's-susceptible mice who were given the equivalent of a human serving of 1–1.5 ounces of walnuts per day showed significant improvement in memory, learning skills, and motor skills and a reduction in anxiety. This result is buttressed by another study that found that walnut extract provided protective benefits against beta-amyloid—a protein that has been found in the brains of those with Alzheimer's disease.

It's not just walnuts that are beneficial for brain health, though. Nuts in general are a rich source of vitamin E, an antioxidant-rich, fat-soluble vitamin that helps protect the brain from damage from free radicals.

Blueberries

Blueberries are the only fruit specifically recommended on the MIND diet. The diet doesn't prohibit the consumption of other fruits, but it also doesn't emphasize increased consumption of all fruits like the Mediterranean and DASH diets. However, blueberries are purposely included in the diet because of their significant brain-boosting power.

Blueberries get their color from a class of compounds called flavonoids. They're especially rich in a specific flavonoid group called anthocyanins. A study published in the journal *Free Radical Biology & Medicine* in 2004 reported that the flavonoids in blueberries are able to cross the blood-brain barrier and interact with the nerve cells (neurons) in the brain, improving communication between the neural networks and stimulating the regeneration of new brain cells. This process can improve both short-term and long-term memory and help increase the ability to retain new information. According to the researchers involved in the study, these discoveries have major implications for both the prevention and treatment of Alzheimer's disease.

In another study, this one performed on aging rats, researchers at Tufts University found that when compared to rats on a controlled, standard diet, rats that were fed blueberries performed better on memory, coordination, and balance tests. Although this was an animal study, researchers point out that improvements in humans could be similar, and if so, it would improve quality of life as you age.

FACT

Anthocyanins are members of the bigger flavonoid group called phytochemicals. They are responsible for the deep blue color of blueberries and are also found in açaí, bilberries, cherries, red grapes, and purple corn. In addition to their anti-inflammatory effects, anthocyanins have also been shown to reduce the risk of cancer and protect heart health.

Another study published in the *Journal of Agricultural and Food Chemistry* found that after twelve weeks of supplementation with wild blueberry juice, older adults who had begun to experience slight memory problems showed improvement in learning and recall abilities than adults who did not consume blueberry juice. In addition, the anthocyanins in blueberries in particular help move blood into the areas of the brain that are responsible for memory and learning.

Whole Grains

The ability of whole grains to help ward off Alzheimer's disease comes mainly from their fiber content. Whole grains are rich in fiber, which helps slow the digestion and absorption of food through your digestive tract. When digestion is slowed down, it also slows down the release of glucose in your blood. As a result, you don't experience a rapid surge in blood sugar— or the rapid surge in insulin levels that follows.

If your body consistently experiences dramatic increases in blood sugar and insulin, over time it can lead to insulin resistance—a condition in which the body is unable to use insulin effectively. Research shows that insulin resistance could increase the risk of developing Alzheimer's disease by changing the way your brain uses glucose—or sugar—which is its preferred source of energy. When you become insulin resistant, glucose cannot enter the cells effectively, and as a result, your brain—and other parts of your body—can become starved of energy.

Whole grains also contain a wide variety of B vitamins and other vitamins and minerals that work together to reduce inflammation, combat oxidative stress, and reduce blood pressure—three factors that play a role in the development of brain and heart diseases.

Beans

Beans and other legumes, like green peas, are rich in B-complex vitamins, which protect the brain against shrinkage and help to maintain a healthy nervous system. Like whole grains, beans are also rich in fiber, so they can help slow down digestion and keep blood sugar and insulin levels steady.

Fish

Fatty fish, like salmon, are especially high in omega-3 fatty acids. These fatty acids help protect the brain against beta-amyloid—the protein whose presence is linked to higher incidences of Alzheimer's disease. A study published in *Archives of Neurology* found that people aged sixty-five and older who ate at fish at least twice a week for a period of at least six years had a 13 percent decrease in loss of cognitive functioning when compared to adults of the same age who didn't eat fish regularly. Adults who ate fish at least once a week for a period of six years experienced a 10 percent reduction in cognitive decline.

ESSENTIAL

There is circumstantial evidence that heavy metals, like mercury, might cause or at the very least exacerbate the symptoms and progression of Alzheimer's disease. To avoid unnecessary exposure to mercury, choose low-mercury fish that are high in omega-3 fatty acids, such as salmon, tilapia, cod, and catfish.

Although the fatty acids in fish are powerful, the benefits don't end there. Fish is also rich in vitamin B_{12}, which helps counteract the effects of homocysteine, an amino acid that, at high levels, contributes to many diseases, including Alzheimer's disease, heart failure, and age-related macular degeneration.

Poultry

Poultry products, like chicken and turkey, are rich in a B vitamin called nicotinamide—or vitamin B_3—that proves promising for reversing memory loss and cognitive decline in those with Alzheimer's disease. Like most intervention studies, the study that brought this information to light was an animal study published in the *Journal of Neuroscience*. Researchers genetically engineered mice to develop the equivalent of human Alzheimer's disease. Then they gave the mice an amount of vitamin B_3 that was equivalent to a human getting 2–3 grams. The mice that were treated with the vitamin supplement showed a complete reversal of symptoms, and when given a series of cognitive tests they performed as though they were never afflicted by the disease at all. The creators of the MIND diet took into account the significance of this study when determining the amount of poultry to include in the diet to provide the body with vitamin B_3.

Olive Oil

Olive oil is one of the foundations of both the Mediterranean diet and the MIND diet. It has been well documented that olive oil is good for the heart, but more recently, after seeing reduced rates of Alzheimer's disease and dementia in those following a Mediterranean-style diet, researchers have become interested in how olive oil may also be good for your brain.

ESSENTIAL

A study out of the University of California–Davis found that many commercial extra-virgin olive oils are actually a combination of cheaper, less healthy oils and may contain no real extra-virgin olive oil at all. When purchasing an olive oil, make sure to choose one from a reputable source.

Some of the benefits of olive oil on brain health are due to its abundance of antioxidants and monounsaturated fats. Research has shown that heart-healthy unsaturated fats can protect blood vessels all over the body—including those in the brain, which in turn helps reduce the damage that can contribute to Alzheimer's disease and other forms of dementia. Other studies, however, look closely at a specific compound in olive oil called oleocanthal. Researchers have found that oleocanthal may help speed up the removal of beta-amyloid, a protein in the brain that has been linked to Alzheimer's disease, preventing it from forming the gummy plaques in the brain that are associated with Alzheimer's disease. Oleocanthal does this by increasing the production of proteins and enzymes that are necessary to carry beta-amyloid out of the brain.

Red Wine

Red wine is a staple among the people of the Mediterranean area, and although excess alcohol consumption is never recommended, researchers have concluded that drinking one to three glasses of red wine per day may not only be good for heart health but may improve brain health as well.

ALERT

A note about alcohol: Studies have shown that a moderate intake of red wine (no more than one glass per day for women or two glasses per day for men) may have protective benefits for the brain and heart. That being said, if you do not drink alcohol, it's not necessary to incorporate it into your plan to experience results.

Red wine contains resveratrol—a phenolic compound that is found primarily in the skin of grapes. In preclinical studies, resveratrol has been shown to have numerous biological functions that can protect the body from neurodegenerative diseases, like Alzheimer's, as well as cancer and heart disease. In one small study, Dr. R. Scott Turner, a professor of neurology and director of the Memory Disorders Program at Georgetown University, and his team studied a group of 119 men and women for a period of one year. The group was split in half—with one half given 1,000 milligrams of resveratrol daily for a year and the other half given a placebo. After the year was over, Dr. Turner and his colleagues looked at the study participants' brains and assessed their cognitive level.

The participants who were given resveratrol showed no buildup of beta-amyloid protein in the brain, while the participants on the placebo showed the accumulation of the protein, as is typical of Alzheimer's patients. In addition, the group taking resveratrol showed fewer signs of inflammation and injury in the brain and showed slight improvements in their ability to take care of themselves, such as getting dressed for the day or bathing themselves.

Herbs and Spices

All herbs and spices are allowed on the MIND diet plan, and you should take advantage of them. Herbs and spices not only provide flavor to your dishes, but some of them have brain-boosting power. For example, curcumin, the active ingredient in turmeric, has been shown to reduce inflammation in the brain and help break up the plaques in the brain associated with Alzheimer's disease. Cinnamon increases the levels of compounds called neurotrophic factors in the brain. These compounds help stimulate the birth of new neurons, protect existing neurons, and protect the brain from neurodegenerative disorders. Research shows that even just smelling cinnamon may have these brain-protective factors. Sage helps boost memory, thyme increases the amount of DHA in the brain, rosemary decreases cognitive decline in people with dementia, and garlic promotes better blood flow to the brain. Get creative with your spices. Vary them and try new things; just make sure to always read your labels. Some herbs and spices are highly processed and may contain things like hydrogenated vegetable oils. Before using or purchasing a spice, look at the ingredient list to make sure that the actual spice is the only ingredient.

Weekly Menu

In an effort to make the diet plan easy to follow, there are no strict rules for exactly what you can eat and how you eat it, but your weekly menu should look something like this: Each day, you'll consume three servings of whole grains, a salad, another vegetable (that's not considered a leafy green), and a glass of wine. On most days, you'll snack on a small amount of nuts, and every other day you'll include a serving of beans. You will include poultry, like chicken or turkey, and a ½ cup of berries at least twice per week. Fatty fish, like salmon, will be your main course at least once per week, and you'll do all your cooking in olive oil. When you have a salad, it's beneficial to use olive oil as your dressing.

One of the charms of the MIND diet is that, unlike other complicated diet plans, there are no specific macronutrient—protein, fat, and carbohydrate—percentages that you must adhere to. If you're following the program as written and consuming the recommended amount of each type of food, you'll naturally get the macronutrients you need. While following the plan, most of your calories will come from carbohydrates, followed by fat, and then protein.

ESSENTIAL

Typically, while following the MIND diet, carbohydrates will provide 50–60 percent of total calories, fat will provide 25–35 percent of calories (with fewer than 8 percent of these calories coming from saturated fat), and the rest—15–25 percent of calories—will come from protein.

Unhealthy Food Categories

The five food categories on the brain-unhealthy list are not expressly forbidden, but it's recommended to limit them or avoid them as much as possible. The diet recommendations are as follows:

- Red meat—less than four servings per week
- Butter/margarine—less than 1 tablespoon per day
- Cheese—less than one serving per week
- Desserts, sweets, and added sugar—less than five servings per week
- Fried food and/or fast food—less than one serving per week

Think of these guidelines for the brain-unhealthy foods as upper limits. What that means is that you don't have to consume the amounts listed per day and/or week; it means that's the absolute most that you can have. For example, if you avoid red meat completely, that's great; if you decide to have red meat, you cannot exceed four servings per week.

There are good reasons for the exclusions of these foods, and many are related to each other. Let's take a look at the benefits of excluding these foods and the other benefits that the MIND diet can help you achieve . . .

CHAPTER 3

Additional Benefits of the MIND Diet

When you focus on a diet that's rich in anti-inflammatory, antioxidant-rich foods and devoid of foods that largely contribute to weight gain and inflammation, you'll begin to notice an improvement in all areas of your health. The MIND diet was developed to improve brain health and reduce the risk of Alzheimer's disease and other neurodegenerative disorders, but following the program results in other health benefits as well. In this chapter you'll learn all about the MIND diet's benefits and how they can help protect your brain and reduce your risk of experiencing cognitive decline.

Improving Your Blood Sugar and Insulin Levels

Your blood sugar levels, or the amount of the simple sugar glucose and the hormone insulin in your blood at any given time, have a major impact on your health. In the short term, low blood sugar levels can present as blurry vision, increased heartbeat, mood changes, nervousness, pale skin, headache, hunger, increased sweating, skin tingling, and shaking. If blood sugar levels get too low, it can even result in fainting or loss of consciousness. The initial symptoms of high blood sugar levels include dry mouth, thirst, frequent urination, blurry vision, dry/itchy skin, fatigue, weight loss, and increased appetite. Over time, high blood sugar levels can also lead to insulin resistance, and if left uncontrolled for an extended period of time can cause Type 2 diabetes, a condition characterized by the body's inability to effectively control blood sugar levels on its own, and/or metabolic syndrome, and can even have a detrimental effect on brain function.

FACT

Your brain prefers glucose as its primary source of energy. Tight regulation of glucose in the blood is essential to ensure that your brain is working properly. When glucose and insulin levels get out of whack, your brain is often the first organ to become negatively affected. While other tissues can turn to fat for energy, your brain begins to feel starved.

Insulin is a hormone produced by your pancreas that plays a central role in allowing your body to use the food you eat as energy. When you eat carbohydrates, your body breaks them down into glucose, a form of sugar that your body uses (and your brain prefers) for energy. The glucose enters your bloodstream and your pancreas releases insulin in response. Insulin's job is to carry glucose into your cells. Some is used up right away, and the rest is converted to glycogen and stored in your liver for later use as energy in between meals. As insulin carries glucose out of your bloodstream, your blood sugar levels go back down. In a healthy person, this process allows both insulin and glucose to stay within normal ranges.

Insulin Resistance and Metabolic Syndrome

Most experts agree that there are a variety of factors involved in developing insulin resistance, but the key underlying causes are excess weight (especially in the stomach area), physical inactivity, inadequate sleep, and poor diet. Insulin resistance is a condition in which the pancreas produces insulin, but the muscle, fat, and liver cells do not respond to it properly. As a result, glucose builds up in the bloodstream, signaling the release of more insulin. If the pancreas can keep up with this overproduction of insulin, glucose and insulin levels will remain normal. If it continues, eventually the pancreas will not be able to keep up, and glucose will continue to build up. This can lead to diabetes, prediabetes, and other serious health problems like metabolic syndrome.

Metabolic syndrome is not a specific disease but rather the name for a group of risk factors that raise your risk of heart disease and other health conditions like diabetes and stroke. The following five risk factors are defined as metabolic risk factors: a large waistline, a high triglyceride level, a low "good" cholesterol level, high blood pressure, and a high fasting blood sugar level. In order to be diagnosed with metabolic syndrome, you must present with at least three of the five risk factors.

Decreased Brain Function and Alzheimer's Disease

Past studies have implicated both Type 1 and Type 2 diabetes as contributors to Alzheimer's disease, but newer research shows that it might not just be diabetes that's a factor but high blood sugar itself. Researchers from the Washington University School of Medicine in St. Louis published a study in the *Journal of Clinical Investigation* that reported that any situations in which blood sugar levels are not properly controlled can have detrimental effects on brain function and speed up the progression of degenerative neurological conditions like Alzheimer's disease.

Their animal study found that injecting glucose into the bloodstream of mice prompted the brains of the mice to increase their production of beta-amyloid. In fact, a doubling of glucose levels in the blood caused beta-amyloid production to increase by as much as 20 percent. After these findings, the team repeated the procedure on older mice that already had Alzheimer's disease–related plaque in their brains and found that the same doubling of glucose levels in the blood led to a whopping 40 percent increase in beta-amyloid production. What this means is that high, uncontrolled blood glucose levels are damaging on their own, but they can be even more detrimental for people who already have symptoms of Alzheimer's disease.

The MIND Diet and Blood Sugar and Insulin Levels

The types of foods that affect your blood sugar levels the most are refined, rapidly digesting carbohydrates, like white breads, white crackers, white rice, potatoes, sweets, and desserts. The more processed a sugar is, the faster it moves through your digestive system and into your bloodstream. The faster that sugar moves through your digestive system, the more dramatic the resulting spike in blood sugar is. The MIND diet eliminates these foods and encourages the consumption of slower-digesting carbohydrates like berries, beans, lentils, green leafy vegetables, and nuts. These foods are not only inherently good for your brain; they also help stabilize your blood sugar and insulin levels. Other ways you can keep your blood sugar and insulin levels steady include eating three balanced meals and small snacks throughout the day, avoiding skipping meals, and avoiding overeating.

Achieving Healthy Cholesterol Levels

Research shows that a high level of cholesterol in the blood is linked to an increased risk of Alzheimer's disease because cholesterol is thought to play a role in the creation of beta-amyloid, the protein linked to the disease. The MIND diet limits the foods that play the biggest role in increasing bad cholesterol levels and decreasing good cholesterol levels, like red meat, cheese, fried foods, and sweets, which often contain trans fats—the worst offender of all.

In addition to removing cholesterol-forming foods, the diet also encourages eating fiber-rich foods like vegetables, berries, whole grains, nuts, and beans that promote healthy cholesterol levels. Dietary fiber, which is the part of the plant that is not broken down during digestion, is found exclusively in plant-based foods.

High-Cholesterol Foods

Red meat, butter, and cheese contain a high ratio of saturated fat to unsaturated fats and a significant amount of dietary cholesterol. In metabolic studies, foods with this type of fat profile typically led to a poor blood cholesterol profile—or high levels of LDL, which is often called "bad cholesterol," and low levels of HDL, which is referred to as "good cholesterol." Trans fats, like those found in fried foods and many commercial baked sweets and pastries, have a particularly noticeable negative effect on cholesterol levels.

Although researchers aren't entirely sure why, there is a large amount of evidence that a high blood cholesterol level is related to the development of Alzheimer's disease. Many experts believe it has something to with the fact that cholesterol is involved in both the creation and the placement of the protein beta-amyloid. In one study published in *Neuroepidemiology*, researchers assessed 444 Finnish men. They found that high cholesterol levels in midlife were associated with a threefold increase in Alzheimer's disease later in life. Two other animal studies found that rats and mice that were fed high-fat and high-cholesterol diets showed impairment in learning and a decrease in memory performance compared to animals on a controlled diet. They also experienced other Alzheimer's-related symptoms like deposits of beta-amyloid plaque in the brain and a loss of healthy brain nerve cells.

ALERT

The current recommendation is to consume no more than 2 grams of trans fat per day. The average American adult consumes 5.6 grams daily. Trans fat is so harmful that some states, like New York and Philadelphia, have already passed laws that prohibit restaurants from using any ingredients that add trans fats to their dishes.

Trans fat seems to be the biggest area of concern. According to a study published in *Archives of Neurology*, even a moderate intake of trans fat was shown to increase a person's risk of developing Alzheimer's disease by two to three times when compared to someone who avoided the unhealthy fat.

Fiber-Rich Foods

It may seem as though fiber may not be very beneficial because your digestive system can't break it down, but in addition to keeping your bowels regular, it also helps remove excess cholesterol from your bloodstream. It works like this: A specific type of fiber, called soluble fiber, binds to bile, the liquid that is produced by the liver and helps you digest fat, in the intestines. Normally, after bile is released from the liver, it is re-absorbed once it gets to the small intestine, but when it's attached to fiber, bile is excreted from the body in your feces. The drop in the amount of bile signals the liver to make more. Because the body needs to use cholesterol to make bile, the cholesterol floating around in your bloodstream is reduced as a result. The more fiber you eat, the more bile that is excreted, and the more cholesterol your body needs to make.

FACT

Bile is composed mainly of cholesterol, bile acids (also called bile salts), and bilirubin (a waste product of the breakdown of red blood cells). It also contains small amounts of water, potassium, sodium, copper, and other metals. Bile is produced by the liver and stored in the gallbladder until your body is ready to use it. When you eat a meal that contains fat, your gallbladder releases bile into the small intestine.

The National Academy of Sciences recommends that men eat 38 grams of fiber per day and women consume 25 grams daily. Right now, the average American only takes in 15 grams per day, well below the recommended amount. The MIND diet optimizes fiber intake by encouraging the consumption of several different types of fiber-rich foods, such as whole grains and vegetables, at every meal.

Fish

Fish, which is a staple of the MIND diet, also has cholesterol-lowering properties due to its high concentration of the fatty acids EPA and DHA. Fish obtain these fatty acids by eating phytoplankton, which are rich in omega-3s, and then storing them in their own body fat. That's why fatty fish, like salmon, are often recommended as a first choice. These fatty acids don't just improve cholesterol; they prevent irregular heartbeat, reduce inflammation, lower blood pressure, and decrease triglyceride levels.

Benefiting Your Heart

Research shows that Mediterranean-style diets, the type of diet on which the MIND diet is based, can significantly reduce the risk of heart disease. The focus of the diet isn't necessarily on limiting total fat intake (although you should pay some attention to how many calories you're taking in), but rather paying attention to the types of fats you're eating. Olive oil is rich in monounsaturated fats that help lower cholesterol levels, but it is also high in antioxidants that help protect your heart—and the rest of your body.

The omega-3 fatty acids in the fish recommended on the MIND diet also help promote healthy blood clotting, reduce triglyceride levels, and improve the health of your blood vessels. They are also associated with a decreased incidence of sudden heart attacks.

Strengthening Your Immune System

Your diet plays an integral part in strengthening your immune system—or weakening it if you're eating the wrong types of foods. Research shows that eating a diet high in fruits, vegetables, and whole grains, and low in saturated fats, is one of the first lines of defense against sickness. Certain nutrients are especially good at boosting your immune system, and each one of these nutrients is found in abundance on the MIND diet.

Vitamin C

Leafy green vegetables, like spinach and kale, are loaded with vitamin C—an immune-boosting, water-soluble vitamin. Specific immune cells, called phagocytes and T cells, need vitamin C to fight off foreign invaders and keep you from getting sick. In addition to leafy greens, vitamin C is also found in large amounts in bell peppers and Brussels sprouts.

Vitamin E

T cells are a specific type of white blood cell that are the forefront of the immune response. T cells recognize a foreign invader and send instructions to the rest of your immune system on how to properly attack it. Some T cells recognize and kill virus-infected cells directly, while others help B cells, another type of immune cell, make antibodies—proteins that keep your immune system strong. Vitamin E helps immature T cells form into mature T cells that are able to properly regulate your immune system. Vitamin E is found mainly in foods that contain fat, including avocados, nuts, seeds, olive oil, and wheat germ. Some dark leafy greens and fish also contain vitamin E. These are all staples of the MIND diet.

Vitamin D

Researchers have discovered that vitamin D is critical to immune system activation and that without sufficient intake of vitamin D the T cells are not able to react properly to fight off infection. Unfortunately, the vast majority of Americans are deficient in vitamin D without even realizing it. A large reason for this is that there aren't a lot of foods rich in the vitamin, and the foods that are rich in vitamin D are often undereaten. Rich sources of vitamin D include salmon, mackerel, tuna, and sardines—all of which are included as a foundation on the MIND diet.

Selenium

Selenium is a powerful antioxidant that affects various aspects of human health, including your immune system. The mineral stimulates development and promotes proper functioning of all types of white blood cells, and it enhances the ability of lymphocytes, a certain type of white blood cell, to fight off infection. Rich sources of selenium include broccoli, sardines, tuna, Brazil nuts, and garlic.

Zinc

Research shows that zinc plays a central role in the immune system. It is well documented that people who are deficient in zinc tend to be more susceptible to a wide variety of pathogens that can cause sickness. The presence of zinc is crucial for normal development and function of neutrophils, the most abundant type of white blood cell in mammals. In fact, neutrophils make up 40–75 percent of the white blood cells in your body. The richest dietary sources of zinc include oysters and poultry.

Reducing Inflammation

When your cells are in distress or under some sort of perceived attack, they release chemicals that alert the immune system that they need help. The immune system then sends out its first line of defense—inflammatory cells—in an effort to either heal the wounded tissue or trap the invading substance and kick it out of the body. As this happens, blood vessels release fluid that accumulates at the site of the injury and results in the telltale signs of inflammation—swelling, redness, and pain. When you have a cut or a real immune problem, inflammation is a very important defense mechanism that your body uses to keep you safe and healthy. However, if your immune is overactive, or responding to a more subtle, long-term threat, like a bad diet, inflammation can become chronic and cause a whole host of problems.

When Inflammation Becomes Chronic

When inflammatory cells remain in blood vessels for too long, it promotes the buildup of plaque, which is made up of cholesterol, fatty substances, cellular waste products, calcium, blood-clotting factors, and other substances, that can impede proper blood flow. This is the same plaque that contributes to heart attack and heart disease. The body sees this plaque as a threat and sends out even more inflammatory cells, which only exacerbates the problem. Your body is not equipped to deal with this prolonged and unfocused immune attack, and eventually these inflammatory cells start damaging your internal cells and the other cells in your body. Chronic inflammation is not only associated with an increased risk of developing Alzheimer's disease (because it puts stress on the brain and can damage brain cells); it's also linked to cancer, heart disease, depression, allergies, and diabetes, to name a few.

Stress is another major factor in chronic inflammation. When you're under an extreme amount of stress, your body perceives that stress as an imminent attack and sends out inflammatory cells in response. If you're able to get your stress levels under control, your body will call off the attack and inflammation will subside; however, if stress levels remain high, the attack will become chronic and so will the inflammation.

Increase Magnesium Intake

Your diet can play a significant role in the amount of inflammation in your body. What you eat can either fuel inflammation or cool it down. The foods that are discouraged from the MIND diet, like red meat, sweets (sugary foods), and fried foods, are highly inflammatory foods, while the foods that are the foundation of the program are anti-inflammatory. Some of the main components of the diet, dark leafy greens, nuts, and whole grains, are especially good for reducing inflammation in the body because they are all rich in magnesium—a mineral that an estimated 60 percent of Americans are deficient in. Research shows that people with high inflammatory markers tend to have low levels of magnesium. There also seems to be a connection between low magnesium and inflammation-related disorders like heart disease and diabetes.

Reducing Stress

Research shows that reducing your stress levels can in turn reduce inflammation. In a study published in *Psychosomatic Medicine*, researchers reported that women who practiced 75–90 minutes of hatha yoga twice per week for at least two years had significantly lower levels of C-reactive protein (CRP) and interleukin-6, two markers of inflammation, than women who practiced less frequently.

Dr. Janice Kiecolt-Glaser, professor of psychology and psychiatry at the Institute for Behavioral Medicine Research at Ohio State University College of Medicine, adds that practicing regular yoga doesn't make stress go away; it just changes the way your body responds to stress physiologically. In other words, yoga allows you to handle—and recover from—stressors more easily.

Many people think of getting a massage as a luxury, but it's actually very beneficial for reducing inflammation. Research shows that just one 45-minute massage can lower levels of hormones that promote inflammation by increasing the amount of white blood cells so they can fight them off. A massage can also lower stress hormones, which in turn decreases inflammation.

Balancing Digestive Health

More than 2,000 years ago, Hippocrates, regarded as the "father of medicine," said that all disease begins in the gut. Back then, most health professionals may not have known exactly what he meant by that, but recent research shows that if your gut—or digestive tract—isn't healthy, it's nearly impossible for the rest of you to be healthy.

After all, your body constantly rebuilds and repairs its cells from the nutrients you obtain from food. Your gut is also home to trillions of bacteria. These bacteria ensure proper digestion, but they also play a major role in your immune system and your brain health. Recent research even goes so far as to say that the gut may be the initial place that chronic inflammation begins.

FACT

> Your digestive tract is the site at which all nutrients are absorbed into your bloodstream; it's also the system that determines what goes into your body (via the small intestine) and what is kicked out (through your waste). As you can imagine, these are two very powerful jobs and the cornerstone to the way you feel.

There are many things that challenge the health of your digestive system: poor diet; stress; toxic chemicals in processed foods, water, and personal-care products; overuse of antibiotics; and overconsumption of alcohol. As your digestive system becomes taxed, you may begin to experience a number of uncomfortable symptoms:

- Acid reflux
- Runny nose
- Gas and bloating
- Skin problems/rashes
- Diarrhea or constipation
- Negative reactions to food

If not taken care of, poor digestion can eventually lead to nutrient deficiencies and chronic inflammation. Research has tied unhealthy digestion and gut issues to chronic problems like food allergies, autoimmune diseases, diabetes, chronic infections, depression, and anxiety.

Keys to Healthy Digestion

The first step to balancing your digestive system is to remove any foods or drinks that could be inflammatory or irritating. The next step is to allow your body to start repairing itself by giving it all of the nutrients it needs to build new, healthy cells. By following the MIND diet, you've already got these first two steps covered. You'll also want to make sure you're drinking enough water to keep you hydrated and your digestive system healthy. For many people, these three steps alone are enough to get the digestive system back on track. For others, supplementation may be necessary. Supplements that are especially good for the digestive system are probiotics and digestive enzymes.

Probiotics

The number of bacteria cells in your gut outnumbers your "human" cells by ten to one. In fact, that actually makes you more bacteria than human. Your gut is often coined your second brain because these bacteria play incredibly significant roles in your brain health. Your gut is also where approximately 70 percent of your immune system resides. The bacteria in your gut modulate your inflammatory response. If the balance of gut bacteria is off, it can result in the chronic, widespread inflammation that is associated with Alzheimer's disease and other neurodegenerative disorders like Parkinson's disease and multiple sclerosis.

ALERT

Although probiotics and digestive enzymes are generally considered extremely safe, it's always a good idea to discuss any new supplements with your doctor or a qualified nutritionist before taking them. Your healthcare provider can give you dosage recommendations based on your specific circumstances.

There are several things, like a poor diet and high stress levels, that can throw your gut bacteria out of whack. The key to re-establishing your gut health, and your health in general, is to replenish the "good" bacteria so that it can rebalance the bad. That's where probiotics come in.

Probiotics are live organisms that reinoculate your gut and help maintain a healthy intestinal flora. You can get probiotics into your diet by consuming fermented foods like kimchi, sauerkraut, and kombucha, or you can take a probiotic supplement. If you go the supplement route, choose one that contains several different strains of bacteria and has few to no added fillers.

Digestive Enzymes

Digestive enzymes are natural compounds produced in the body that assist in the breakdown and absorption of nutrients. If your body doesn't contain enough digestive enzymes to support proper digestion, you won't be able to absorb the nutrients you're eating no matter how healthy your diet is. If you experience symptoms like bloating, pain, or belching after meals, it may be necessary to include a digestive enzyme supplement in your regimen.

When choosing a digestive enzyme, look for one that contains several different types. For example, protease helps break down protein, while lipase helps break down fat. Since your meals typically contain a balance of these macronutrients, it's best if your digestive enzyme does too.

Importance of Water

The average human adult body is composed of 50–65 percent water. Water is considered one of the most essential elements because you could survive weeks without food but only a couple of days without water. Drinking an adequate amount of water helps your body remove waste through perspiration, urination, and defecation. Water also helps prevent you from becoming constipated by softening your stools and helping fiber expand so that it can help move food through your digestive tract.

ALERT

Tap water, and even bottled water, can be contaminated with toxic chemicals, heavy metals, and even remnants of prescription medications or drugs that have been flushed down the toilet. It's best to get all of your water from a clean source. You can install a filter on your sink or get a carbon filter that sits in your refrigerator.

Water isn't just important for a healthy digestive system, though; it also plays roles in nutrient transport, detoxification, temperature regulation, and neural communication. Your brain consists of nearly 75 percent water, so water is especially important for proper brain function and the communication of your nervous system.

There is a general rule that you should drink eight 8-ounce glasses of water per day, at minimum, although more recent recommendations suggest that you take your body weight in pounds, divide it in half, and then drink that many ounces. That means if you weigh 150 pounds, you would need 75 ounces of water per day. Of course, because every person is different, your exact water needs depend on your age, sex, size, and activity level, but these general recommendations are a good place to start.

CHAPTER 4

How to Be Successful on the MIND Diet

It doesn't matter how great any diet plan is; the only way that you'll experience success on a particular diet is if you're able to follow it properly. A list of the foods to avoid and the foods to include is essential, but it doesn't always give you all the tools you need to succeed. In this chapter, you'll learn how to incorporate mindful eating and food tracking into your daily life. You'll also learn strategies for meal planning, saving money when shopping, and for identifying (and avoiding) foods that may seem healthy, but aren't. This chapter also provides tips on how to stay satisfied and how to stick to the MIND diet plan while eating out, so that you don't have to miss out on social situations and gatherings. To be successful, you'll have to do a little planning, but with the right tips and tricks, sticking to the MIND diet will become second-nature . . . and you'll even start to enjoy it.

Eating Mindfully

When you hear the word "mindfulness," eating may not be the first thing that comes to mind, but the practice can be enormously beneficial during mealtime. In general, mindfulness describes the practice of being present in the moment. Mindful eating—also referred to as intuitive eating—describes a way of eating in which you really focus on and pay attention to your food, rather than hurrying to get through a meal or eating surrounded by distractions. Mindful eating is about slowing down, savoring your food's flavor and texture, and taking the time to appreciate the food that's on your plate and in your mouth and the nourishment that it's giving your body.

Benefits of Mindful Eating

Research shows that in addition to simply forcing you to slow down, mindful eating has a number of benefits for both your mind and your body. Mindful eating reduces stress, improves digestion, and boosts satisfaction during and after meals. Mindful eating can also decrease overeating and snacking and promote weight loss or the maintenance of a healthy body weight. People who regularly practice mindful eating also report increases in feelings of appreciation for food. When you eat mindfully, you tend to appreciate the food as nourishment rather than as an afterthought.

FACT

According to recent statistics, approximately 20 percent of American meals are eaten in the car while on the go. Only one-third of Americans say they take a break at work for lunch, and 65 percent eat lunch at their desk while continuing to work.

When preparing your own meals, mindful eating starts from the time you begin to prepare the food and ends when you're done with the meal. The core principles of mindful eating include being aware of the nourishment food offers you while you're preparing your meal and while you're eating it; choosing foods that are both enjoyable to eat and nourishing for your body; and recognizing real, physical hunger cues and differentiating them from the desire to eat for other reasons, such as cravings or emotional drivers.

Mindful-Eating Tips

When you're just starting out, it can be difficult to get the hang of mindful eating—especially if you're used to rushing through a meal, eating in your car on the way to work, or sitting down in front of the television for dinner. Fortunately, there are many different things you can do to incorporate mindful-eating practices into your routine until you find the combination that works best for you. Some examples of how to be mindful when you eat include:

- Turn off the television and put away all electronic devices while you eat.
- Before eating, take note of how hungry you are; rate it on a scale of 0 to 10. When you rate your hunger, you can make conscious decisions of how much food you should be eating. If you're really hungry, you may want regular size portions, whereas if your hunger rates on the lower end of the scale, a snack-sized portion may be your best bet.
- Put the fork down between each bite.
- Take time to notice the color and smell of your food before you eat.
- Put a small amount of food in your mouth, but don't chew it for 30 seconds. Instead, pay attention to the flavor and the texture.
- Chew each bite thoroughly and adequately before swallowing.
- Pay attention to how your body feels as you eat: Are you getting full? Do you feel joy or satisfaction from eating the food?
- When you notice yourself start to feel satisfied, stop eating. Don't attempt to finish the entire plate if you're full; save it for later.

Mindful eating is an extremely beneficial practice to incorporate into your life, especially when you're starting a new plan like the MIND diet. Mindful eating allows you to appreciate food as nourishment, which then acts as a driver to make the necessary changes that are required to keep you healthy and your body happy.

Tracking and Journaling Foods

Tracking and journaling foods may seem like a lot of work, but in the long run it can actually save you time—and money. A food journal is particularly helpful on the MIND diet because it can help you keep track of your food intake for the day and the week so you can make sure that you're hitting your daily and weekly recommended servings of the ten brain-healthy food groups. If you meal plan in advance, it also decreases stress because you'll know exactly what you're eating and when, and you'll have a clear overview of how many servings of each group you're taking in. You won't have to scramble at the end of the day or at the end of the week to meet the serving recommendations.

How to Keep a Food Journal

There is no right or wrong way to keep a food journal or to make a meal plan. Your strategy may be different based on your schedule and what methods of organization work best for you, but typically tracking and journaling foods looks something like this:

On Sunday (or a day of the week when you have a couple of uninterrupted hours), sit down and write out what you intend to eat for the entire week. Use the recommended servings from the MIND diet's ten brain-healthy foods list to plan your meals to make sure that you're getting in all the recommended servings. Once your meals are planned out, create a shopping list.

FACT

When creating a shopping list, it's helpful to divide that shopping list into grocery store sections. For example, list all the produce together and all the meat together, so you don't have to scramble through the list while you're at the store to make sure that you have everything.

After you shop and prepare your foods, keep track of what you're eating during the week. Since you've already planned out your meals, try to stick as close to your meal template as possible. Make a new page for every day and write down what you ate, how much you ate, what time it was, and how you felt. If you eat something that's not on your plan, even if it's one bite of a cookie, write that down, too. This isn't about failure or guilt or judgment; the goal with a food journal is to give you an accurate picture of what you're eating and how it's making you feel. No one has to see the food journal except you.

Because the MIND diet is not a calorie-counting program, it's not necessary to count calories as part of your food journaling—unless weight loss is a major goal for you, as discussed later on in this chapter. As long as you're sticking to the recommended servings (and actually eating what's considered a true serving), you'll naturally be consuming the amount of calories your body needs.

Tips for Stress-Free Planning and Shopping

When you're starting a new lifestyle, there must be some level of understanding that you're going to have to make changes. At first these changes may come as a struggle, but eventually they become your way of life. The good news is that there are ways that you can reduce the stress these changes can cause, especially when in the grocery store.

Unhealthy "Healthy" Foods

One of the best stress-free shopping tips is this: Don't waste time trying to find processed foods that fit into your plan. One of the beautiful things about the MIND diet is that it's chock-full of whole foods (foods that are unprocessed and come directly from nature, like fruits, vegetables, and lean meats) and practically devoid of any processed foods. The diet is designed like this for a reason: Whole foods are full of nutrients that contribute to brain health and the health of your entire body, and processed foods tend to be stripped of valuable nutrients and contribute little more than unnecessary calories. You may get lucky and find processed foods that contain ingredients that are on the approved food lists for the MIND diet, but don't waste your time and energy searching for these. Instead stick to these major sections in the grocery store: produce, meat (poultry), oils, beans, and whole grains. If you accept that you're going to be eating only whole foods, your grocery trips will be streamlined and take up much less time.

Saving Money

The MIND diet focuses on a few dietary staples: whole grains, green vegetables, and beans. These are all items that you can generally buy in bulk, and doing so will save you both time and money. You'll probably be able to find chicken and wine at your bulk-food store or in the bulk-food section of a regular grocery store, as well.

Keep It Simple

When starting a new diet plan, it's easy to get overexcited about all the new possibilities and the new foods you're eating, but take a minute to step back and look at your meal plans. Do you have a different meal planned for every single day of the week, or do you incorporate some of the same food items so that you can cook in bulk or eat leftovers for lunch? Try to plan your meals so that you can cook in large quantities. This way, you'll be able to spend less time cooking, shopping, and preparing meals.

The MIND Diet and Weight Loss

The MIND diet wasn't designed with weight loss as the primary goal, but you can certainly lose weight while following the program. If you're currently eating a lot of fried foods, processed foods, desserts, and red meat, you'll likely lose weight just by cutting those foods out and focusing on leaner, clean whole foods; however, if the diet isn't too far off from what you're doing now, you may need to incorporate calorie counting into your plan.

Calorie Counting on the MIND Diet

Calorie counting used to be a lot of work and extremely time-consuming, but thankfully, newer technology has practically taken all the guesswork out of it. There are several online programs and even apps that you can download right to your smartphone that help you determine how many calories you need for the day—both to maintain and/or to lose weight—and help you track the calories you're actually eating. The programs will tell you if you're over or under for the day and will even allow you to log your exercise, which will have an impact on your total calorie deficit.

FACT

Research shows that people who keep a food journal tend to lose more weight than those who don't. When trying to lose weight, many people underestimate exactly how much food and how many calories they're taking in. A food journal forces you to look at your daily intake honestly and gives you an accurate picture of what you're doing.

The foods on the MIND diet are so common and readily available that most food-tracking programs will already have the information for them. All you have to do is determine your calorie needs, track your daily food intake, and then adjust your diet accordingly based on your specific goals.

Feeling Satisfied While Losing Weight

Another bonus to the MIND diet is that it's not a low-fat, low-carbohydrate program that will leave you feeling ravenous and deprived all the time while trying to lose weight. Because the program incorporates lots of healthy fats, you'll feel fulfilled even if you have to cut calories.

So if you're eating a salad, toss some beans on top and drizzle it with olive oil. Add a slice of avocado to your chicken breast and eat it with a side of quinoa. The key is to incorporate some carbohydrates, protein, and fat at every meal to keep you satisfied.

ESSENTIAL

Fat is the most calorie-dense of the three macronutrients: fat, protein, and carbohydrates. Each gram of fat contains 9 calories, while each gram of protein and carbohydrates contains 4 calories. Because it's so calorie-dense, it's extremely filling, but remember to watch your portion sizes because those calories can add up quickly.

Managing Social Gatherings and Dining Out

Attending social gatherings, especially when they're centered around food, and dining out are often the most challenging aspect of sticking to a new eating plan. Typically, meals at social gatherings are not prepared with food restrictions in mind, and restaurants often use inexpensive and easily accessible ingredients that may not be part of your plan. Restaurants are also known for adding in less-than-healthy ingredients to otherwise healthy dishes to boost flavor. Attending social gatherings and dining out while following the MIND diet is not impossible, but it does take a little more preparation. At first this may seem like a challenge, but eventually you'll adapt to your new way of life. The good news is that the MIND diet is meant to be easy to follow, and it allows a little bit of flexibility so that you can indulge every once in a while during these events without guilt or feeling like you've completely veered off track from your plan.

Dining Out

Most restaurants will serve the foods that are recommended on the MIND diet, but it's always a good idea to do your research before you get there. Look up the restaurant's menu online and choose a meal that works for your plan. If you can't find anything you can eat directly off the menu, call the restaurant and ask to speak to the manager or a head chef. Inform him or her that you are on a specific diet plan and ask if the restaurant would be able to accommodate your needs. In most cases, the restaurant will be happy to follow your requests, especially if they can put together a meal with everything they have on hand. And with the wide variety of foods allowed on the MIND diet, that will be easy enough.

Ask Your Server Questions

Most restaurants will have chicken and a vegetable side or a salad with chicken and dressing on the menu, but unfortunately, there may be hidden ingredients like butter or sugar in these items. If you see something you'd like on the menu, don't be afraid to ask your server questions to double-check the ingredients. If there are ingredients in the dish that you don't want, politely ask that those ingredients be left out of the preparation. Instead of the dressing that comes with a salad, ask for olive oil and balsamic vinegar on the side and make your own dressing. The MIND diet is meant to be flexible and easy to follow, and that includes the times when you're eating out.

Preparing for Social Gatherings

There are two types of social gatherings: ones where you might have a say in the food presented (where you know the host or hostess really well or where you may be invited as a guest of a guest), or ones where you have no say over the food choices (like a large work event). There are ways to prepare for both.

In the first circumstance, one where you know the host or hostess well, speak up before the event. Inform your host that you're following the MIND diet and ask what's on the menu for the night. This will allow you to gauge whether or not there will be something there that's on your plan. If not, it's not necessary to request that a special meal be made; instead, ask your host if he or she is okay with you bringing a side dish to complement the meal. This will give you the opportunity to ensure that there will be something at the event that you can comfortably eat. Good options for a side dish include quinoa loaded with vegetables or maybe a large leafy green salad with avocado and olive oil dressing. In the case of a work event or a situation where you don't know the host, eat before you go. If you attend an event satisfied from your meal, you'll be less likely to veer off track.

Maintaining a Balanced Diet for Life

The MIND diet is not a fad diet or a quick weight-loss plan; it's a way of life. The people who see the most significant results from following the plan are the people who stick to the recommendations as written and follow the diet plan the longest. That being said, following the MIND diet plan doesn't mean that you'll never eat fried food or have a dessert ever again; it just means that you understand that these types of foods are a treat, and you become more mindful of how much of them you're eating and how they make you feel.

In order for a diet to become a way of life, you have to enjoy it and it has to be easy enough for you to incorporate into your lifestyle. The benefits of the MIND diet are just that: The plan is simple and consists of foods that are commonly found, easy to prepare, and taste delicious. At first, adjusting to the MIND diet may be difficult, especially if the way you eat now is a far cry from the recommendations on the plan, but as you get into a groove, you'll find that the program is both simple and enjoyable.

CHAPTER 5

Lifestyle Recommendations for Long-Term Success

There's a reason for the old adage "you are what you eat." The proper nutrition that you get from following the MIND diet is a major part of not just your brain health but the health of your entire body. That being said, the best way to ensure lasting success on the diet—and to experience the greatest results—is to focus on all the areas that make you a human, not just one. That doesn't mean that you have to completely overhaul your entire life overnight. It just means that you should address all the areas of health—mental, physical, emotional, and spiritual—a little at a time. In this chapter, you'll learn how to take care of your body holistically, by practicing self-care, engaging in regular exercise, and practicing mindfulness exercises like yoga and meditation.

The Value of Self-Care

In order to be the best you that you can be, you have to practice self-care. This means taking the time to listen to your body and engage in the things that your body needs to stay healthy. Self-care may involve yoga, journaling, reading a book, meditation, or drawing. It may mean taking some time every day to go for a walk or spend some time in nature.

ESSENTIAL

Self-care doesn't look the same for everyone, but the thing that it has in common in all circumstances is it makes you feel good. It gives you that time to unwind and de-stress—two things that are very important to your brain.

Self-care typically extends beyond yourself, too. Research shows that those who regularly practice self-care have better relationships not only with themselves but with others too.

Responding to Stress and Reducing Stress Levels

In normal amounts, stress is a good thing. In fact, it's what has allowed humans to survive and evolve to become what we are today. Back in caveman times, when a man faced a tiger, his body sent out a surge of adrenaline, noradrenaline, and cortisol that signaled him to do one of two things—run or fight. This response, called the fight-or-flight response, is what kept him alive. If you didn't have this ingrained response to take some type of action, you would get mauled.

The fight-or-flight response is still useful today—it alerts you when there's danger lurking; however, in today's fast-paced modern world, many people are walking around with their fight-or-flight responses chronically activated due to an overloaded work schedule, poor diets, and other life stressors, such as finances. Over time, this prolonged stress response can do a number on your body.

The Mechanics of the Fight-or-Flight Response

The fight-or-flight response, also referred to as the "acute stress response," was brought to light in the 1920s by Walter Cannon. While studying animals, Cannon discovered that their nervous system responds in a very specific way to threats. He then realized that this response was not exclusive to animals but applied to all vertebrates and other organisms.

FACT

There are two parts to your nervous system: the parasympathetic nervous system and the sympathetic nervous system. The sympathetic nervous system is responsible for the body's fight-or-flight response and prepares the body for intense physical activity. The parasympathetic nervous system is responsible for the body's rest-and-digest response; it relaxes the body and slows down high-energy functions.

When a person experiences a threat, whether that threat is real (like a lion in your path) or perceived (like worrying about paying the bills), the body responds by triggering the sympathetic nervous system. The sympathetic nerves release a substance called acetylcholine that prompts the adrenal glands to release adrenaline and noradrenaline (or norepinephrine) and cortisol. The release of these hormones causes increases in both the heart rate and breathing rate and constricts blood vessels. It also causes the eyes to dilate (to allow you to see more clearly) and slows digestion, so all blood and energy can move to your limbs (in case you need to run for your life). Normally, when the threat goes away, the hormones level out, the neurons stop firing, and the parasympathetic nervous system takes over again, allowing you to go back into a state of relaxation. When you're under chronic stress, there is a constant release of adrenaline, noradrenaline, and cortisol into the blood. It may not be the same rapid surge that occurs in a life-threatening situation, but the constant, unwavering exposure can wreak havoc over time.

Chronic Stress

In a study published in 2014, neuroscientists at the University of California–Berkeley demonstrated that chronic stress can actually trigger long-term changes in both brain structure and function such as changes in volume of gray matter versus white matter and destruction of neurons. When neurons are destroyed, it can affect your memory in negative ways. Chronic stress can also slow down the production of new brain cells, create fear and anxiety, make you more emotional, deplete levels of feel-good neurotransmitters like serotonin, and disrupt your ability to think clearly and make rational decisions.

In addition to its physical effects on the brain, chronic stress can also affect the musculoskeletal, respiratory, cardiovascular, endocrine, gastrointestinal, and reproductive systems. The effects are extremely far-ranging and can be disastrous. Some possible effects of chronic stress include muscle tension, headaches, difficulty breathing, rapid heart rate, high blood pressure, heartburn, constipation or diarrhea, decreased sexual desire, and changes to menstruation cycles. Chronic stress is also linked to widespread, chronic inflammation, which is a factor in many of today's health problems.

Managing and Reducing Stress

Stress is inevitable, especially in this modern world. It would be impossible to completely get rid of all stress. The realistic goal is not to avoid stress entirely but to find ways that allow you to manage or respond to stress in healthier ways. There is not a "one-size-fits-all" approach to stress reduction; it's about finding things that work for you. However, some things that have proven wildly successful in reducing stress include proper nutrition (like that recommended on the MIND diet), regular exercise and yoga, a regular and adequate sleep schedule, a healthy social life, and meditation and mindfulness.

Meditation and Mindfulness

Meditation and mindfulness seem to be the talk of the town lately, but they aren't anything new. In fact, some of the earliest written records of meditation go as far back as 1500 B.C. Meditation and mindfulness are commonly used as a way to quiet the mind and reduce stress levels, but their benefits go way beyond this. A regular mindfulness meditation practice can literally change the structure of the brain.

While meditation and mindfulness are two terms that go hand in hand, they're not entirely the same. The definition of meditation is spending some time in quiet thought, while the definition of mindfulness is the state of being aware or conscious of the particular moment. Many people incorrectly think that in order to meditate "correctly" you must clear your mind and have no thoughts, and that to be mindful you must be able to go with the flow and let nothing bother you, but that's not exactly how it works.

Contrary to popular belief, the goal of meditation is not to become free of thought but to acknowledge a thought, let it pass, and then return to the present moment. The same holds true for mindfulness: If a thought pops into your head, acknowledge it, let it go, and then come back to the present moment. The goal isn't to avoid the thought but to not let it carry you away into a downward spiral of worry or stress.

Meditation and the Brain

In 2013, researchers at the Beth Israel Deaconess Medical Center specifically looked at how meditation may be able to help those with Alzheimer's disease and those at risk of developing Alzheimer's disease and other neurodegenerative conditions. They divided fourteen adults between the ages of fifty-five and ninety into two groups. One group received traditional care, but with no emphasis on meditation. The other group engaged in meditation and yoga for at least two hours every week, in addition to receiving traditional care. Researchers found that the group who engaged in yoga and meditation had less degeneration in their brains and experienced better brain connectivity than the control group.

Other brain-boosting benefits of meditation have also been demonstrated in various studies. Researchers have found that meditation can:

- Protect the brain by increasing protective tissues
- Help reduce feelings of loneliness and isolation (two feelings that can increase the risk of developing Alzheimer's disease)
- Reduce perceived stress and evoke feelings of calm
- Reduce the stress hormone cortisol, which, when uncontrolled, has been shown to increase the risk of developing Alzheimer's disease
- Increase gray matter and thickness of the cortex, which may slow the rate at which the brain ages

Those who meditate regularly also appear to have less degeneration in the area of the brain called the hippocampus, which plays important roles in both short- and long-term memory. People with Alzheimer's disease tend to have a shrunken hippocampus. Meditation has also been shown to reduce levels of inflammatory proteins in the body. Chronic inflammation is not only tied to Alzheimer's disease but many other chronic diseases.

A Simple Mindfulness Exercise

Find a comfortable chair, couch, or bed—you can even do this sitting up on the floor or standing if you'd like—and sit or lie down comfortably. If you are sitting in a chair, sit up straight and feel the way the chair supports your back and your buttocks. If you are lying down, pay attention to the sensations of the bed and how it feels in the areas where it meets your body. If you are standing, make sure you maintain good posture and notice the way your feet feel touching the floor. Take some deep breaths in through your nose and out of your mouth, and notice how your stomach expands as you breathe.

ESSENTIAL

When you're taking deep breaths, your breath should expand your abdomen, not your chest. If you experience most of the expansion in your chest, your breaths are too shallow. Imagine your abdomen as a balloon and allow it to fill up with air as you breathe.

As you do this, you will probably notice some thoughts popping into your head. That's okay. Picture your thoughts like waves in the ocean. Let them come to you and then let them float away. As you're breathing, you can also do a body scan. Start at the top of your head and slowly work your way down; notice any sensations or discomfort and slowly relax your muscles as you go. Let your forehead become loose, make sure your tongue and jaw are loose and slightly open, and continue your way down the entire length of your body until you reach your toes.

Start out by doing this exercise for 5–10 minutes each day, then work your way up to at least 20–30 minutes. It's a good idea to engage in a mindfulness practice right after you wake up, while you're still lying in bed, before you start your day.

Starting and Maintaining an Exercise Routine

Although exercise isn't a specific recommendation on the MIND diet, starting and maintaining an exercise routine is one of the best things that you can do for your health. Exercising regularly doesn't just improve your brain function and mental clarity; it reduces your risk of chronic disease, improves balance and coordination, contributes to weight loss, improves your sleep, and boosts your self-esteem and confidence levels.

Exercise and the Brain

Exercise, both directly and indirectly, improves memory and thinking. In fact, Dr. Laura Baker, an associate professor of gerontology and geriatric medicine at the Wake Forest School of Medicine, describes regular aerobic exercise as a "fountain of youth" for the brain. Directly, exercise reduces inflammation, improves insulin resistance, and stimulates the release of growth factors—chemicals in the brain that affect the health of existing brain cells, the growth of new blood vessels in the brain, and the creation and survival of new brain cells. Indirectly, exercise helps improve mood and allows you to sleep better, which then improves thinking, memory, and concentration.

Several studies show that the prefrontal cortex and medial temporal cortex—the parts of the brain that control thought and memory—are larger in people who exercise regularly when compared to people who don't exercise. Dr. Maria Carrillo, the chief science officer for the Alzheimer's Association, adds that regular exercise plays a role in both protecting your brain from Alzheimer's disease and other forms of dementia and in improving quality of life if you're already affected by the disease.

Getting Started

When starting a new exercise routine, the first thing you want to do is get clearance from your doctor that you're healthy enough to exercise. Once that's done, it's time to design a fitness program that works for you. It's easy to say that you're going to start exercising every day, but will you stick to that plan? If you don't exercise at all now, start with a smaller goal—maybe three to four times per week, then work your way up. When designing your routine, it's also important to consider your goals. Are you trying to lose weight?

Are you incorporating exercise to reduce stress levels? That will make a difference not only in the type of exercise you should choose but how often you'll need to exercise to experience the results you're looking for. Once you decide on your goals, adopt a routine that fits into your schedule. Make sure that you're doing enough to experience benefits, but that you're not pushing too hard right out of the gate. The Mayo Clinic recommends that most adults should engage in at least 150 minutes of moderate-intensity exercise per week.

One of the best ways to ensure that you'll stick to your new exercise routine is to make sure that you're choosing exercises and activities that you like. If you hate to run, don't rely on the treadmill for exercise. The point is not to suffer through it; it's to enjoy the process. Find something you enjoy. There are plenty of options out there. You can find a group fitness class, join a sports team or a running club, or find a workout buddy to partner up with. You can even try a lower-impact exercise, like yoga, to get you started.

The Benefits of Yoga

Like meditation, yoga is a practice that has been around for centuries but is more recently coming to the forefront as a way to combat stress, anxiety, and symptoms of serious conditions, such as arthritis and fibromyalgia. Yoga is a combination of physical movement and postures and meditation and controlled breathing. On a physical level, yoga can increase flexibility and strength, elongate and tone the muscles, and provide a fantastic stretch, but that only touches the surface of its benefits.

A study performed at the University of Illinois found that just a 20-minute session of yoga can improve focus and the ability to retain new information. Other research shows that yoga can boost mood, reduce anxiety and inflammation, and lower stress levels.

Yoga also:

- Increases muscle strength
- Improves your posture
- Protects your spine
- Contributes to bone and joint health
- Increases blood flow
- Boosts immunity

- Drains your lymphatic system
- Lowers blood sugar
- Improves balance
- Helps you sleep better
- Increases self-esteem

There are many different styles of yoga and many different levels—from beginners to advanced. If you're just starting out, it can be helpful to take a beginner's class with a certified instructor who can show you the proper way to hold your poses and teach you the right breathing technique.

Fostering a Sense of Purpose

Having a sense of purpose means having a direction in life—feeling like you're doing something meaningful in life and making a difference in the world or the lives of others. According to research published in *Psychological Science*, a sense of purpose may help you live longer, no matter your age or your current health status. Some people are lucky enough to find their sense of purpose at a young age, while others don't have that a-ha moment until much later in life. It doesn't matter how old you are; it's never too late to find your purpose in life.

Benefits of a Sense of Purpose

Fostering a sense of purpose is an important aspect of protecting the brain and preventing Alzheimer's disease. After studying thousands of elderly subjects, Dr. Patricia Boyle, a neuropsychologist at the Rush Alzheimer's Disease Center, found that people with a low sense of life purpose were almost two and a half times more likely to develop Alzheimer's disease than those with a strong sense of purpose.

In addition to protecting your brain and just making you feel better in general, having a sense of purpose may also protect against heart disease and allow you to deal with pain more effectively. Those with a high sense of purpose also tend to have better relationships because they give more time and attention to their loved ones and are more engaged and active in those relationships. There is also strong evidence that those with a sense of purpose are better able to handle and adapt to the ups and downs of life. They have an increased ability to "go with the flow" because they feel like no matter what roadblocks arise, they are on a meaningful path.

How to Find a Sense of Purpose

Finding a sense of purpose isn't always easy—and it can look different for everyone—but in general, there are some things that those who find their sense of purpose have in common. Usually, the commonality is that a sense of purpose is something that extends beyond the self and has an ability to affect others. It could be a service that you offer or something creative that you share with the world. It could be something as simple as spreading love and kindness wherever you go. The key is to find the things that make you happy, the things that make you feel like your life is meaningful. What is it that you do in your spare time? What gets you out of bed in the morning? These are the things that will give you clues as to how you can foster your sense of purpose.

The Importance of Sleep

Sleep is a necessity. It's one of your basic human needs, and yet many people treat sleep as a luxury rather than a priority. There has been extensive research done in the area of sleep, and across the board, experts agree that both sleep quality and quantity have a major impact on your health.

In the United States, four out of ten Americans admitted to getting fewer than seven hours of sleep per night. Nearly 30 percent of these adults reported getting even fewer than six hours of sleep each night.

After a single night of poor sleep or a night when you've slept for fewer than six hours, your cognitive throughput—or the speed at which your brain processes information—slows down. This is because poor-quality sleep disrupts the neural pathways that allow different areas of your brain to communicate with each other. After a couple of nights of no or poor sleep, your hormone levels begin to fluctuate, which affects your hunger response. You may feel hungry when you're not and have a harder time feeling full when you do eat. Your brain also has trouble making and sorting new memories and has a harder time staying focused and eliminating distractions when you're tired.

If you go weeks without adequate sleep, neurons in your brain begin to die off and proteins that normally would have been cleared away during sleep begin to accumulate in the brain. The accumulation of these proteins can lead to problems with attention span and processing information. Those who are chronically sleep deprived are also more likely to develop feelings of depression.

Sleep Recommendations

The National Sleep Foundation has done extensive research on how much sleep people of different ages need in order to function optimally. Their latest recommendations, published in their journal *Sleep Health*, are as follows:

- Older adults (sixty-five and older): 7–8 hours
- Adults (twenty-six–sixty-four): 7–9 hours
- Young adults (eighteen–twenty-four): 7–9 hours
- Teenagers (fourteen–seventeen): 8–10 hours
- School-age children (six–thirteen): 9–11 hours
- Preschool-age children (three–five): 10–13 hours
- Toddlers (one–two): 11–14 hours
- Infants (four–eleven months): 12–15 hours
- Newborns (birth–three months): 14–17 hours

Keep in mind that although too little sleep is a more common issue, getting too much sleep may also have negative effects on your health, concentration, and focus.

Supplements

When following the MIND diet correctly, you should be getting all the protein, fat, carbohydrates, vitamins, and minerals you need to keep your body healthy, but there are some things that are fantastic for your brain that are difficult to get from your diet alone. Supplements aren't required while following the MIND diet program, but they can give you certain compounds that you won't be able to get from food alone. If you're at a high risk of developing neurodegenerative disease, you may want to consider taking some of the following recommended supplements in addition to following the diet plan.

Ginkgo

Studies show that ginkgo may be beneficial for cerebral insufficiency—a condition in which there is a decreased blood flow to the brain due to clogged blood vessels. Researchers believe that ginkgo works by thinning the blood, which improves oxygen flow to the brain. An increase in oxygen to the brain can result in improved memory as well as improved attention span and can reduce your risk of memory-related disorders. Some research also suggests that ginkgo may be as effective as certain classes of drugs for early-stage Alzheimer's disease.

Ginkgo is available in tablet, tea, and capsule form—and the amounts used in scientific studies typically range from 80–240 milligrams in divided doses during the day. Ginkgo is generally safe, but it does have some blood-thinning properties, so if you're considering taking it as a supplement, make sure to discuss it with your doctor first.

Citicoline

Citicoline is a naturally occurring compound that's found in every cell of your body. Research shows that supplementation with citicoline may increase blood flow to the brain, help build healthy cell membranes, increase brain plasticity (or the ability to learn and retain new information), and boost the brain's energy by providing support to the cells' mitochondria. It may also increase levels of dopamine, which is the neurotransmitter responsible for motivation and productivity, and acetylcholine, which is involved in memory and learning.

Curcumin

Curcumin is the active ingredient in the spice turmeric. While you can get curcumin from adding turmeric to your food, it's also often available in supplemental form because it's so powerful. Curcumin is classified as anti-inflammatory, antiviral, antibacterial, antifungal, and anticancer. It's also a powerful antioxidant. Curcumin boosts brain power by reducing inflammation in the brain and breaking up the plaque that is associated with Alzheimer's disease. It also increases levels of dopamine and serotonin—the neurotransmitter responsible for feelings of happiness. Although curcumin is powerful, it's not readily absorbed by the body—in fact, 85 percent of the curcumin you take in gets excreted. Consuming curcumin with piperine, a compound found in black pepper, can increase its absorption rate by up to 2,000 percent, so if you're looking for a supplement, it's a good idea to find one that contains both compounds.

CHAPTER 6

Breakfast

Perfect Vegan Pancakes

These vegan pancakes are dairy- and egg-free, which makes this dish cholesterol-free as well. But the taste and texture? It's all there! Light, fluffy, dreamy, steamy, and delicious, these pancakes are perfect. If you're watching your fat, omit the oil.

PREP TIME: 5 minutes
COOK TIME: 20 minutes

INGREDIENTS | SERVES 4

1⅓ cups white whole-wheat flour
¼ cup beet sugar
2 tablespoons ground flaxseed
1 tablespoon baking powder
6 tablespoons water
1 tablespoon vanilla extract
2 tablespoons olive oil
1⅓ cups almond milk

What Is Flaxseed?

Flaxseed, also known as linseed, is a healthy source of omega-3 fatty acids, fiber, and antioxidants. It has a mild, slightly nutty flavor and is often sold in ground form, making it easy to add to a variety of dishes. Ground flaxseed can be used successfully as an egg substitute in many baked goods. Simply stir 1 tablespoon ground flaxseed with 3 tablespoons water for each egg you'd like to replace, then set aside 5 minutes to thicken. Once thickened, add to the recipe as you would the egg/s.

1. Measure flour, sugar, flaxseed, and baking powder into a medium mixing bowl and whisk well to combine.

2. Add the remaining ingredients and stir until incorporated.

3. Heat a nonstick griddle or medium skillet over medium-low to low heat. Once hot, ladle roughly ⅓ cup batter onto the hot pan. Cook until bubbles appear on the surface of the pancake and the bottom is golden brown, roughly 2–3 minutes. Flip the pancake and cook 2–3 minutes more, then remove pancake from heat. If pancakes brown too quickly, lower heat to low.

4. Repeat cooking process with remaining batter. Serve pancakes warm.

PER SERVING Calories: 290 | Fat: 9.5 g | Protein: 6.3 g | Sodium: 420 mg | Fiber: 6.3 g | Carbohydrates: 48.2 g | Sugar: 15.3 g

Lemon Poppy Seed Pancakes

*These Lemon Poppy Seed Pancakes are your favorite citrus muffin—
in pancake form! For the brightest flavor, use the juice and zest of
1 fresh lemon as the recipe describes, but 2 tablespoons lemon juice
and ½ teaspoon lemon extract can be substituted in a pinch.*

PREP TIME: 5 minutes
COOK TIME: 20 minutes

INGREDIENTS | SERVES 4

¾ cup unbleached all-purpose flour

½ cup white whole-wheat flour

¼ cup sugar

1 tablespoon baking powder

1 tablespoon poppy seeds

Grated zest and juice of
1 medium lemon

1 cup almond milk

1 tablespoon agave nectar

1 tablespoon olive oil

2 teaspoons vanilla extract

1. Measure flours, sugar, baking powder, poppy seeds, and lemon zest into a medium mixing bowl and whisk together. Add remaining ingredients and whisk until combined.

2. Heat a nonstick griddle or medium skillet over medium-low to low heat. Ladle roughly ¼ cup batter onto the hot pan. Cook until bubbles appear on the surface of the pancake and the bottom is golden brown, roughly 2–3 minutes. Flip the pancake and cook 2–3 minutes more, then remove pancake from heat. If pancakes brown too quickly, lower heat to low.

3. Repeat cooking process with remaining batter. Serve pancakes warm.

PER SERVING Calories: 264 | Fat: 5.2 g | Protein: 5.1 g | Sodium: 406 mg | Fiber: 3.5 g | Carbohydrates: 50.5 g | Sugar: 18.6 g

From Soup to . . . Pancakes?

Soup ladles aren't just for soup. They work wonderfully for measuring and pouring pancake batter onto any hot cooking surface. The resulting pancakes will be perfectly shaped and sized, and you'll never have to worry about messy cleanup!

Gingerbread Pancakes

*Ground ginger, cinnamon, cloves, a little brewed coffee,
and brown sugar flavor these scrumptious vegan pancakes,
creating a holiday-worthy breakfast you can enjoy year-
round. Serve warm, drizzled with pure maple syrup.*

PREP TIME: 5 minutes
COOK TIME: 20 minutes

INGREDIENTS | SERVES 4

1¼ cups white whole-wheat flour

¼ cup brown sugar

1 tablespoon baking powder

2 teaspoons ground ginger

1 teaspoon ground cinnamon

⅛ teaspoon ground cloves

1 cup almond milk

¼ cup brewed coffee, cooled

2 tablespoons olive oil

2 teaspoons vanilla extract

1. Measure flour, brown sugar, baking powder, ginger, cinnamon, and cloves into a medium mixing bowl and whisk until all lumps are gone.

2. Add remaining ingredients and whisk well to combine.

3. Heat a nonstick griddle or medium skillet over medium-low to low heat. Ladle ¼ cup batter onto the hot pan. Cook until bubbles appear on the surface of the pancake and the bottom is golden brown, roughly 2–3 minutes. Flip the pancake and cook 2–3 minutes more, then remove pancake from heat. If pancakes brown too quickly, lower heat to low.

4. Repeat cooking process with remaining batter. Serve pancakes warm.

PER SERVING Calories: 256 | Fat: 7.9 g | Protein: 5.4 g | Sodium: 409 mg | Fiber: 5.5 g | Carbohydrates: 44.7 g | Sugar: 13.7 g

Peanut Butter and Jelly Pancakes

Fresh from the griddle, these vegan pancakes taste just like a warm whole-wheat peanut butter and jelly sandwich. Top the light and fluffy batter with sliced banana or fresh blueberries for an extra-special treat. Strawberry jam is just a suggestion; any flavor of fruit jam may be substituted instead.

PREP TIME: 5 minutes
COOK TIME: 20 minutes

INGREDIENTS | SERVES 4

1¼ cups white whole-wheat flour
2 tablespoons sugar
1 tablespoon baking powder
3 tablespoons peanut butter
3 tablespoons strawberry jam
1¼ cups almond milk
1 tablespoon vanilla extract

Almond Milk and Other Nondairy Alternatives

The MIND diet limits the consumption of dairy products, including cow's milk, so almond milk is used throughout the recipes in this book for consistency. Its creamy, mild taste and wide availability make it a great stand-in for traditional milk. Almond milk is sold in both sweetened and unsweetened forms, either plain or vanilla-flavored. Look for it in the refrigerated dairy section of most supermarkets or in sealed shelf-stable packaging elsewhere in the store. An equal amount of another non-dairy milk (soy, rice, coconut, hemp, or oat) may be substituted for the almond milk in any recipe in this book.

1. Measure flour, sugar, and baking powder into a medium mixing bowl and whisk well to combine.

2. Add remaining ingredients and stir until incorporated.

3. Heat a nonstick griddle or medium skillet over medium-low to low heat. Ladle roughly ¼ cup batter onto the hot pan. Cook until bubbles appear on the surface of the pancake and the bottom is golden brown, roughly 2–3 minutes. Flip the pancake and cook 2–3 minutes more, then remove pancake from heat. If pancakes brown too quickly, lower heat to low.

4. Repeat cooking process with remaining batter. Serve pancakes warm.

PER SERVING Calories: 290 | Fat: 6.8 g | Protein: 8.3 g | Sodium: 478 mg | Fiber: 6.1 g | Carbohydrates: 51.8 g | Sugar: 17.1 g

Homemade Vegan Sausage

This homemade vegan sausage is flavored with an array of herbs and has a subtle pepper kick. The recipe yields 12 (2") patties, enough to feed 6. It's better tasting than commercial vegetarian sausage and so much better for you, too!

PREP TIME: 20 minutes
COOK TIME: 5 minutes

INGREDIENTS | SERVES 6

1 tablespoon ground flaxseed
3 tablespoons water
¾ cup quick oats
2 tablespoons white whole-wheat flour
2 tablespoons nutritional yeast
1½ teaspoons ground sage
1½ teaspoons onion powder
1 teaspoon brown sugar
½ teaspoon cumin seeds
½ teaspoon dried marjoram
½ teaspoon fennel seeds
½ teaspoon garlic powder
¼ teaspoon freshly ground black pepper
⅛ teaspoon dried thyme
⅛ teaspoon ground rosemary
1 tablespoon low-sodium soy sauce
2 tablespoons olive oil, divided
1 cup cooked brown rice

1. Place ground flaxseed and water in a small bowl and stir to combine; set aside.

2. Place oats, flour, nutritional yeast, sage, onion powder, brown sugar, cumin seeds, marjoram, fennel seeds, garlic powder, pepper, thyme, and rosemary in a food processor and pulse well to combine.

3. Add soy sauce, 1 tablespoon oil, rice, and flaxseed mixture and pulse until the mixture gathers together in a ball.

4. Remove the mixture from the food processor and separate into 2-tablespoon portions. Roll into balls and press into 2" patties.

5. Heat remaining oil in a large skillet over medium-low heat. Place the patties in the pan and brown 2–3 minutes per side.

6. Remove patties from pan and place on a paper towel to drain. Serve immediately.

PER SERVING Calories: 140 | Fat: 5.8 g | Protein: 3.7 g | Sodium: 89 mg | Fiber: 2.8 g | Carbohydrates: 18.4 g | Sugar: 1.0 g

Maple Turkey Sausage

Perfect for those on the MIND diet looking for a lean breakfast meat, these homemade patties are super speedy, subtly sweet, and absolutely delicious. Feel free to substitute lean ground chicken for the turkey. For another twist on the recipe, instead of forming into patties, brown the mixture along with chopped onion, bell pepper, and garlic and serve with scrambled eggs for a hearty breakfast bowl.

PREP TIME: 10 minutes
COOK TIME: 10 minutes

INGREDIENTS | SERVES 8

2 pounds lean ground turkey

1 egg white

1 tablespoon pure maple syrup

1 tablespoon ground sage

½ teaspoon dried red pepper flakes

½ teaspoon fennel seeds

½ teaspoon freshly ground black pepper

½ teaspoon ground rosemary

¼ teaspoon garlic powder

1. Combine ingredients in a large bowl and mix well using a fork or your hands. (The mixture will be sticky.) Form into 16 (2") patties.

2. Heat a nonstick griddle or medium skillet over medium and brown patties on both sides, about 5 minutes per side. Lower heat to medium-low or low if patties brown too quickly. Drain on paper towels, then serve.

PER SERVING Calories: 138 | Fat: 1.9 g | Protein: 27.3 g | Sodium: 64 mg | Fiber: 0.3 g | Carbohydrates: 2.2 g | Sugar: 1.6 g

Maple Syrup Facts

Maple syrup production begins each spring when maple trees are tapped and their sap collected; each tapped tree yields roughly 5–15 gallons of sap. The collected sap is boiled in large vats until much of the water evaporates, leaving behind a concentrated syrup that is then filtered and bottled. On average, it takes 40 gallons of sap to produce just 1 gallon of syrup! Maple syrup is extremely low in sodium, contains calcium and magnesium, and is prized for its distinctive flavor and sweetness.

Peppery Apple-Chicken Sausage

A delicious change from standard ground chicken, these breakfast patties are studded with sautéed apple, onion, and garlic and have a nice peppery kick. If you prefer less spice, reduce the amount of ground pepper to ¼ teaspoon.

PREP TIME: 10 minutes
COOK TIME: 15 minutes

INGREDIENTS | SERVES 4

1 teaspoon olive oil

1 small onion, peeled and chopped

2 cloves garlic, minced

1 medium apple, peeled, cored, and chopped

1 pound lean ground chicken

1 teaspoon ground sage

1 teaspoon brown sugar

½ teaspoon freshly ground black pepper

¼ teaspoon fennel seeds

⅛ teaspoon dried rosemary

1. Heat oil in a skillet over medium heat. Add onion, garlic, and apple and cook 5 minutes or until soft, stirring occasionally. Remove from heat and set aside to cool.

2. Place chicken, sage, brown sugar, pepper, fennel seeds, and rosemary in a medium mixing bowl. Add cooled apple mixture to chicken mixture and mix well with a fork or your hands. Form into 8 (3") patties.

3. Heat the skillet over medium heat and brown patties on both sides, roughly 5 minutes per side. If patties brown too quickly, lower heat to medium-low or low. Drain on paper towels, then serve.

PER SERVING Calories: 213 | Fat: 9.6 g | Protein: 20.3 g | Sodium: 69 mg | Fiber: 1.4 g | Carbohydrates: 10.8 g | Sugar: 7.2 g

Hearty Whole-Grain Breakfast Bowl

With a little leftover brown rice and some quick oats, there's no excuse for not eating breakfast. This heart-healthy meal comes together in minutes and will keep you satisfied for hours. Filled with whole-grain goodness, chopped nuts, and fruit, it's a delicious way to start any day.

PREP TIME: 2 minutes
COOK TIME: 3 minutes

INGREDIENTS | SERVES 1

¼ cup quick oats

½ cup cooked brown rice

½ cup almond milk

1 tablespoon chopped walnuts

1 tablespoon pure maple syrup

¼ teaspoon ground cinnamon

⅛ teaspoon ground ginger

½ cup fresh blueberries

1. Place oats, rice, milk, nuts, maple syrup, cinnamon, and ginger in a small microwave-safe bowl. Cover tightly with plastic wrap and microwave 3 minutes on high.

2. Carefully remove plastic wrap, stir well to combine, and top with blueberries. Serve immediately.

PER SERVING Calories: 356 | Fat: 7.9 g | Protein: 7.4 g | Sodium: 87 mg | Fiber: 6.4 g | Carbohydrates: 65.9 g | Sugar: 23.7 g

Differences in Oats

Oats come in three main types. Quick or instant oats have been precooked and dried. They have the fastest cooking time and are great for making oatmeal or adding to baked goods. Old-fashioned rolled oats have been put through a steaming process to speed cooking. They're considered all-purpose and work well in most recipes. Steel-cut oats are cut, not rolled. They have a chewy texture that's good for oatmeal and other recipes, but because of their longer cooking time aren't ideal for everything.

Instant Banana Oatmeal

Say hello to your new breakfast buddy! With just 3 ingredients and 3 minutes of your time, this all-natural recipe is low-fat, gluten-free, cholesterol-free, free of refined sugar, high in fiber, and absolutely delicious. Enjoy as is or sprinkle with a dash of ground cinnamon.

PREP TIME: 1 minute
COOK TIME: 2 minutes

INGREDIENTS | SERVES 1

½ cup quick oats
¾ cup water
1 medium ripe banana, peeled and mashed

1. Measure oats and water into a small microwave-safe bowl and stir to combine.

2. Place bowl in microwave and cook 2 minutes on high.

3. Remove bowl from microwave and stir in the mashed banana. Serve immediately.

PER SERVING Calories: 258 | Fat: 2.4 g | Protein: 6.6 g | Sodium: 10 mg | Fiber: 7.2 g | Carbohydrates: 54.4 g | Sugar: 14.8 g

Instant Peaches and Cream Oatmeal

This speedy breakfast makes healthy eating downright enjoyable. Quick oats and canned peaches come together in minutes to create an absolutely delicious meal that'll keep you fueled all morning. The clear-plastic 4-packs of 4-ounce fruit cups sold in many supermarkets are perfect for this recipe.

PREP TIME: 1 minute
COOK TIME: 2 minutes

INGREDIENTS | SERVES 1

½ cup quick oats
¾ cup almond milk
½ cup diced peaches in fruit juice
⅛ teaspoon ground cinnamon

1. Measure oats and milk into a small microwave-safe bowl and stir to combine.

2. Place bowl in microwave and cook 2 minutes on high.

3. Remove bowl from microwave and stir in peaches with juice. Sprinkle with cinnamon. Serve immediately.

PER SERVING Calories: 255 | Fat: 4.1 g | Protein: 6.9 g | Sodium: 127 mg | Fiber: 6.2 g | Carbohydrates: 48.7 g | Sugar: 18.5 g

Eating Right on the Road

Sticking to a healthy diet can be a real challenge when traveling. When staying in a chain hotel that provides free breakfast, skip the meat and eggs and opt for oatmeal instead. You can dress up plain oatmeal with fresh, dried, or canned fruit; a small packet of fruit preserves or peanut butter; or a sprinkling of brown sugar. Oatmeal is high in vitamin A, iron, and calcium, and is a good source of protein and fiber. It's a simple meal that will keep you full without compromising your health.

Two-Potato Hash Browns

With these Two-Potato Hash Browns a breakfast favorite gets a makeover—and emerges fat-free and fabulous! The prep work for this recipe is a breeze if you have a food processor with a shredder blade. If not, a standard hand grater will work just fine. If desired, sprinkle the hash browns with your choice of seasonings before serving.

PREP TIME: 10 minutes
COOK TIME: 14 minutes

INGREDIENTS | SERVES 4

2 medium potatoes, peeled and shredded

2 medium sweet potatoes, peeled and shredded

1. Place potatoes in a stockpot and fill with water until potatoes are covered by an inch. Let rest 10 minutes.

2. Drain potatoes into a colander, rinse, and press down to remove as much water as possible.

3. Heat a medium nonstick pan or griddle over medium-low heat. Add shredded potatoes to the hot pan. Cook 7 minutes, then flip potatoes over (this may be a bit messy) and cook 7 minutes more.

4. Remove hash browns from pan and serve immediately.

PER SERVING Calories: 112 | Fat: 0.1 g | Protein: 2.7 g | Sodium: 32 mg | Fiber: 2.7 g | Carbohydrates: 26.1 g | Sugar: 2.7 g

Vegetable Hash

This hearty one-pan breakfast filled with a rainbow of sautéed vegetables and beans is a great change from standard brunch fare and is so much healthier, too. Be sure to cut the potatoes into a small dice so they become tender without the other vegetables overcooking. If the hash begins to stick to the pan during cooking, add a tiny bit of water or vegetable broth to the skillet and stir to release.

PREP TIME: 15 minutes
COOK TIME: 25 minutes

INGREDIENTS | SERVES 6

3 tablespoons olive oil

1 large onion, peeled and diced

1 large potato, peeled and diced

1 large sweet potato, peeled and diced

3 cloves garlic, minced

1 medium green bell pepper, seeded and diced

1 medium red bell pepper, seeded and diced

8 ounces fresh mushrooms, sliced

3 cups fresh chopped kale leaves

1 (15-ounce) can black beans, drained and rinsed

2 tablespoons nutritional yeast

1 tablespoon low-sodium soy sauce

1½ teaspoons all-purpose seasoning

1 teaspoon ground paprika

1 teaspoon ground cumin

¼ teaspoon dried oregano

½ teaspoon freshly ground black pepper

1. Heat oil in a large sauté pan over medium heat. Add onion and potatoes and cook 10 minutes, stirring often.

2. Add garlic, bell peppers, and mushrooms and cook 10 minutes, stirring often.

3. Add remaining ingredients to the pan and stir to combine. Cook and stir 5 minutes or until vegetables are tender and kale has wilted.

4. Remove from heat and serve immediately.

PER SERVING Calories: 212 | Fat: 6.9 g | Protein: 9.1 g | Sodium: 191 mg | Fiber: 7.9 g | Carbohydrates: 29.8 g | Sugar: 4.9 g

What Is a Hash?

Hash is a cooked dish in which all of the ingredients are chopped. The word itself comes from the French verb *hacher* (meaning "to chop"). Different types of hash are popular throughout the world and most all of them combine onions and potatoes in some form, often with meat and other seasonings.

Apple, Banana, and Carrot Muffins

These Apple, Banana, and Carrot Muffins are packed with healthy fruit and vegetables. They must be cooled fully before serving; otherwise, they'll stick to the wrapper and resemble something more akin to a bread pudding. The muffins are best consumed the same day they're baked, but leftovers can be wrapped and frozen for freshness.

PREP TIME: 15 minutes
COOK TIME: 25 minutes

INGREDIENTS | SERVES 12

2 teaspoons ground cinnamon

7 tablespoons sugar, divided

2 medium apples, peeled, cored, and chopped

1 cup grated carrot

1 medium ripe banana, peeled and mashed

4 tablespoons olive oil

¼ cup almond milk

1 tablespoon vanilla extract

1¼ cups white whole-wheat flour

½ teaspoon baking powder

1. Preheat oven to 350°F. Line a 12-cup muffin pan with paper liners and set aside.

2. To make the muffin topping, measure cinnamon and 3 tablespoons sugar into a small bowl and whisk well to combine. Set aside.

3. To make the batter, place apples, carrot, and banana in a medium bowl and stir to combine. Add oil, milk, remaining 4 tablespoons sugar, vanilla, flour, and baking powder and stir until just combined.

4. Spoon batter evenly into the muffin cups, then sprinkle cinnamon-sugar mixture evenly over the batter.

5. Place pan on middle rack in oven and bake 20–25 minutes, until tester inserted into center of muffin comes out clean.

6. Remove pan from oven and place on wire rack to cool. Cool fully, then remove muffins from pan and serve.

PER SERVING Calories: 144 | Fat: 4.7 g | Protein: 2.0 g | Sodium: 30 mg | Fiber: 2.9 g | Carbohydrates: 25.3 g | Sugar: 12.8 g

Whole-Grain Strawberry Muffins

The combination of plump, moist strawberries and subtle crunch of cornmeal is irresistible. Let the freshly baked muffins cool at least 10 minutes before serving to ensure the paper wrappers come off with ease.

PREP TIME: 5 minutes
COOK TIME: 20 minutes

INGREDIENTS | SERVES 12

1 cup white whole-wheat flour

½ cup cornmeal

½ cup sugar

1 tablespoon baking powder

1 cup chopped fresh strawberries

1 cup almond milk

3 tablespoons olive oil

2 teaspoons vanilla extract

Strawberry Facts

Prized for their bright red color and sweet taste, strawberries can be enjoyed in every way imaginable, whether eaten fresh, frozen, dried, or preserved. The garden variety grown today was first cultivated in France in the 1700s. Unlike some other species of fruit, strawberries do not ripen after picking, so must remain on the plant until peak ripeness. Strawberries are a great source of vitamin C and manganese, and are believed to reduce the risk of Alzheimer's and many other ailments, including hypertension, inflammation, cancer, and cardiovascular disease.

1. Preheat oven to 375°F. Line a 12-cup muffin pan with paper liners and set aside.

2. Place flour, cornmeal, sugar, and baking powder in a medium mixing bowl and whisk well to combine.

3. Add strawberries, milk, oil, and vanilla and stir until incorporated.

4. Fill muffin cups roughly ⅔ full. Place muffin pan on the middle rack in oven and bake 20 minutes, until tester inserted into center of muffin comes out clean.

5. Remove pan from oven and place on wire rack to cool. Cool at least 10 minutes, remove muffins from pan, and serve.

PER SERVING Calories: 125 | Fat: 3.8 g | Protein: 1.9 g | Sodium: 137 mg | Fiber: 2.0 g | Carbohydrates: 22.0 g | Sugar: 9.7 g

Zucchini Muffins

This recipe is a great way to consume that bumper crop of summer zucchini. These moist muffins are absolutely delicious and freeze beautifully, so you can bake several batches to enjoy in colder weather. After shredding the zucchini, place in a clean dishtowel, twist, and squeeze; you want to remove as much excess liquid as possible before making the batter.

PREP TIME: 10 minutes
COOK TIME: 25 minutes

INGREDIENTS | SERVES 12

1¼ cups shredded zucchini, drained

2 egg whites

⅔ cup sugar

⅓ cup olive oil

2 teaspoons vanilla extract

1 teaspoon ground cinnamon

¼ teaspoon ground nutmeg

2 teaspoons baking powder

1½ cups white whole-wheat flour

¼ cup chopped walnuts

¼ cup seedless raisins

1. Preheat oven to 350°F. Line a 12-muffin tin with paper liners and set aside.

2. Place zucchini in a medium mixing bowl and add egg whites, sugar, oil, vanilla, cinnamon, and nutmeg. Stir well.

3. Add baking powder and stir. Add flour, walnuts, and raisins and stir just until combined.

4. Divide batter evenly between muffin cups. Place pan on middle rack in oven and bake until tester inserted in center comes clean, about 25 minutes.

5. Remove muffin pan from oven and place on wire rack to cool. Cool at least 10 minutes, remove muffins from pan, and serve.

PER SERVING Calories: 178 | Fat: 7.7 g | Protein: 3.2 g | Sodium: 91 mg | Fiber: 2.5 g | Carbohydrates: 26.3 g | Sugar: 13.4 g

Blueberry Lemon Cornbread

Subtly sweet and dotted with juicy blueberries, this Blueberry Lemon Cornbread makes a delicious breakfast or anytime treat. The basic recipe works equally well with other berries, especially blackberries, raspberries, or chopped strawberries. Either fresh or frozen berries may be used, but frozen berries must be thawed and drained before adding. If you prefer muffins, pour batter into a standard 12-muffin tin and bake at 400°F for 25 minutes.

PREP TIME: 5 minutes
COOK TIME: 30 minutes

INGREDIENTS | SERVES 16

1 teaspoon plus ½ cup olive oil, divided
1 tablespoon ground flaxseed
3 tablespoons water
1 cup almond milk
1 teaspoon lemon juice
1 cup white whole-wheat flour
1 cup cornmeal
¾ cup sugar
1 tablespoon baking powder
1 teaspoon fresh-grated lemon zest
1 cup blueberries (fresh or frozen)
1 teaspoon vanilla extract

Blueberry Facts

Blueberries have been harvested for thousands of years in North America and are an easy garden crop, requiring only acidic soil and adequate rainfall. Blueberries are high in vitamins K and C as well as manganese, and contain several antioxidants believed to inhibit memory loss, cancer, and inflammation. Fresh blueberries make an excellent addition to hot or cold cereals, baked goods, salads, and sauces, but are fairly perishable. To prevent spoilage, freeze blueberries and thaw as needed. Blueberries are also sold dried, like raisins, and make a terrific healthy snack.

1. Preheat oven to 400°F. Lightly oil an 8" square baking pan with 1 teaspoon olive oil and set aside.

2. Combine flaxseed and water in a small bowl and set aside. Pour milk into a measuring glass, add lemon juice, and set aside.

3. Measure flour, cornmeal, sugar, baking powder, and lemon zest into a large mixing bowl and whisk well to combine. Add blueberries to flour mixture and toss gently to coat.

4. Combine flaxseed mixture, milk–lemon juice mixture, ½ cup oil, and vanilla in a small bowl and then add to flour mixture; stir gently until just combined. Do not overmix!

5. Pour batter into prepared pan. Place on the middle rack in the oven and bake 30 minutes, until tester inserted into center comes clean. Remove pan from oven and place on wire rack to cool. Cool 10–15 minutes, then cut into squares and serve.

PER SERVING Calories: 163 | Fat: 7.6 g | Protein: 1.8 g | Sodium: 104 mg | Fiber: 1.9 g | Carbohydrates: 23.3 g | Sugar: 10.8 g

Best Ever Vegan Banana Bread

Irresistibly moist, tender, and bursting with banana flavor, this is hands-down the best banana bread ever. When making banana bread, it's important not to overmix! The batter can become gummy quickly, so measure ingredients into the bowl and stir gently until just combined.

PREP TIME: 10 minutes
COOK TIME: 1 hour 15 minutes

INGREDIENTS | SERVES 20

3 tablespoons ground flaxseed

9 tablespoons water

3 medium ripe bananas, peeled and mashed

1 cup sugar

1½ cups white whole-wheat flour

1 tablespoon baking powder

½ cup olive oil

1 tablespoon vanilla extract

¼ cup chopped walnuts

1. Preheat oven to 350°F. Oil and flour an 8" × 3" loaf pan and set aside.

2. Measure flaxseed and water into a small bowl, stir to combine, and set aside.

3. Place bananas in a large mixing bowl. Add sugar, flour, baking powder, oil, vanilla, nuts, and flaxseed mixture. Stir gently until just combined, then transfer batter to the prepared pan.

4. Place pan on middle rack in oven and bake 1 hour and 15 minutes, until tester inserted into the center comes clean. Remove pan from oven and place on a wire rack to cool.

5. Gently invert pan to remove cooled loaf. Cover loaf or store in an airtight container for up to 3 days.

PER SERVING Calories: 149 | Fat: 6.8 g | Protein: 1.8 g | Sodium: 74 mg | Fiber: 2.1 g | Carbohydrates: 21.7 g | Sugar: 12.3 g

CHAPTER 7

Appetizers and Snacks

Garlicky Steamed Clams

These Garlicky Steamed Clams make a quick and easy appetizer that feels elegant. In this recipe, fresh clams are steamed in a simple white wine broth scented with garlic, lemon, and parsley. If you don't have a fresh lemon, substitute 2–3 generous tablespoons bottled lemon juice instead. Vegetable broth may substituted for the chicken broth, if desired.

PREP TIME: 10 minutes
COOK TIME: 14 minutes

INGREDIENTS | SERVES 4

1 teaspoon olive oil
1 small onion, peeled and chopped
3 cloves garlic, minced
4 tablespoons dry white wine
1 cup chicken broth
Juice and grated zest of
1 medium lemon
¼ cup chopped fresh parsley
½ teaspoon freshly ground black pepper
2 dozen small fresh clams, scrubbed

1. Heat oil in a large sauté pan over medium heat. Add onion and garlic and cook, stirring, 3 minutes. Add wine and stir 1 minute; then add broth, lemon juice and zest, parsley, and pepper.

2. Add clams to the pan and stir well to coat. Cover the pan and steam until clams open, roughly 7–10 minutes.

3. Uncover pan and discard any unopened clams. Serve immediately with remaining broth.

PER SERVING Calories: 122 | Fat: 1.7 g | Protein: 15.5 g | Sodium: 919 mg | Fiber: 0.7 g | Carbohydrates: 7.0 g | Sugar: 1.4 g

Clam Facts

Clams are a type of mollusk with a chewy texture and salty taste. Although naturally higher in sodium than some other seafoods, they can still be a part of a healthy diet. Clams are very low in fat and high in protein, iron, omega-3s, vitamin B_{12}, selenium, and manganese. When buying clams, let your eyes and nose guide you. Fresh uncooked clams should have a mild smell and closed shells. Any open shells should be tapped gently; clams that close can be cooked, and those that stay open are dead and should be discarded.

Mussels in Red Wine

This dish is made up of succulent mussels bathed in a tomato-infused red wine broth. Enjoy this as a starter for any meal, or double the recipe and serve with green salad and whole-grain pasta for a spectacular main course. If you don't have fresh tomatoes and basil, substitute one 15-ounce can of no salt added diced tomatoes and a teaspoon of dried basil instead.

PREP TIME: 10 minutes
COOK TIME: 10 minutes

INGREDIENTS | SERVES 4

1 teaspoon olive oil
1 small onion, peeled and chopped
2 cloves garlic, minced
2 ripe medium tomatoes, chopped
¼ cup dry red wine
¾ cup vegetable juice
3 tablespoons chopped fresh basil
1 teaspoon agave nectar
¼ teaspoon dried thyme
¼ teaspoon freshly ground black pepper
2 dozen fresh mussels, scrubbed and beards removed

1. Heat oil in a large sauté pan over medium heat. Add onion and garlic and cook, stirring, 3 minutes. Add tomatoes and cook, stirring, 2 minutes. Add wine, juice, basil, agave, thyme, and pepper.

2. Add mussels to the pan and stir well to coat. Cover the pan and steam until mussels open, roughly 5 minutes.

3. Uncover pan and discard any unopened mussels. Serve immediately with remaining broth.

PER SERVING Calories: 138 | Fat: 2.7 g | Protein: 12.7 g | Sodium: 357 mg | Fiber: 1.6 g | Carbohydrates: 11.5 g | Sugar: 5.1 g

Spinach and Walnut Stuffed Mushrooms

This dish is a savory treat that is perfect for any occasion. Tender mushrooms are stuffed with a deliciously seasoned mixture of onion, garlic, walnuts, and spinach. Many supermarkets sell packaged "stuffing" mushrooms specifically for this purpose, but any good-sized fresh mushrooms will do. Feel free to vary the nuts and greens for variety: pecans and kale, peanuts and arugula, and so on.

PREP TIME: 10 minutes
COOK TIME: 35 minutes

INGREDIENTS | SERVES 8

16 ounces fresh stuffing mushrooms
¼ cup walnuts
1 small red onion, peeled and quartered
3 cloves garlic

2 cups fresh baby spinach
3 tablespoons bread crumbs
2 tablespoons nutritional yeast
1 tablespoon low-sodium soy sauce
1 teaspoon all-purpose seasoning
1 teaspoon dried basil
½ teaspoon freshly ground black pepper
Olive oil cooking spray

1. Preheat oven to 400°F. Line a baking sheet with parchment and set aside.

2. Gently remove stems from mushrooms and set aside. Arrange mushroom caps stem side up on the baking tray; allow space between caps.

3. Place nuts in a food processor and chop coarsely. Add mushroom stems, onion, garlic, and spinach and pulse to chop finely.

4. Transfer spinach mixture to a medium mixing bowl; add bread crumbs, nutritional yeast, soy sauce, seasoning, basil, and pepper and stir well to combine.

5. Fill each mushroom cap with 1–2 tablespoons filling. Spray the caps lightly with cooking spray.

6. Place the baking sheet on the middle rack in the oven and bake until tender, 35 minutes.

7. Remove from oven and serve immediately.

PER SERVING Calories: 55 | Fat: 2.3 g | Protein: 3.7 g | Sodium: 111 mg | Fiber: 1.5 g | Carbohydrates: 6.2 g | Sugar: 1.7 g

Shrimp with Cocktail Sauce

This dish is a perfect starter for almost any occasion. Double or triple the recipe (or more!) for a party. This works well with either fresh or frozen shrimp, but be sure to thaw shrimp fully before serving. The cocktail sauce is spicy and tangy, almost identical to the store-bought kind, only better! When plating feel free to arrange the shrimp atop a lettuce-lined platter or hang tail-side out from stemmed glasses for added interest.

PREP TIME: 1 hour
COOK TIME: N/A

INGREDIENTS | SERVES 4

½ pound cooked medium shrimp, peeled and deveined

2½ tablespoons tomato paste

1½ tablespoons apple cider vinegar

1½ tablespoons molasses

1 tablespoon horseradish

1 teaspoon ground mustard

1 small clove garlic, grated

1. Place shrimp in a colander and rinse well under cold water. Plate shrimp, cover, and refrigerate until serving.

2. Add tomato paste, vinegar, molasses, horseradish, mustard, and garlic to a small bowl and stir to combine. Cover and refrigerate at least 1 hour, then serve.

PER SERVING Calories: 104 | Fat: 1.1 g | Protein: 13.6 g | Sodium: 634 mg | Fiber: 0.6 g | Carbohydrates: 9.5 g | Sugar: 7.5 g

Shrimp Facts

Shrimp are low in calories, high in protein, and contain many key nutrients, including selenium, vitamin B_{12}, phosphorous, choline, copper, and iodine. Shrimp even contain antioxidants—something rarely found in meat. Shrimp are high in cholesterol, but contain very little saturated fat, making them a healthy part of a MIND diet when eaten in moderation.

Citrus-Marinated Shrimp Cocktail

*A delightful change from classic shrimp cocktail, this refreshing appetizer
will leave you wanting more. Either fresh or thawed frozen shrimp may
be used. Garnish with citrus wedges and fresh cilantro when serving.*

PREP TIME: 3–6 hours
COOK TIME: N/A

INGREDIENTS | SERVES 4

½ pound cooked medium shrimp,
peeled and deveined

⅓ cup orange juice

⅓ cup lemon juice

¼ cup ketchup

1 tablespoon olive oil

1 medium shallot, peeled and minced

1½ teaspoons horseradish

2 tablespoons chopped fresh cilantro

1. Combine all ingredients in a large bowl and mix well. Cover and refrigerate 3–6 hours.

2. Drain and serve.

PER SERVING Calories: 118 | Fat: 4.2 g | Protein: 13.4 g | Sodium: 613 mg | Fiber: 0.5 g | Carbohydrates: 6.6 g | Sugar: 3.7 g

Frozen Shrimp

Much of the "fresh" shrimp sold in supermarkets has been previously frozen and thawed, so don't be discouraged from buying the prepackaged kind. Frozen shrimp is convenient, practical, and economical. To thaw frozen shrimp, place in a colander in the sink and run under cold water for about 5 minutes, tossing periodically to ensure all are defrosting. Test the shrimp by bending gently; once thawed, they will be soft and pliable.

Pan-Fried Calamari

If you love deep-fried calamari, try this healthier homemade version. Fresh or frozen squid is sold in many supermarkets and often comes pretrimmed and cleaned. When cooking, be sure to watch the clock carefully; calamari becomes rubbery if left in the oil for too long.

PREP TIME: 10 minutes
COOK TIME: 10 minutes

INGREDIENTS | SERVES 4

3 tablespoons white whole-wheat flour
1 tablespoon cornmeal
4 large squid tubes (roughly 4 ounces), washed and sliced into ¼"-thick rings
Olive oil for frying
Juice of 1 medium lemon

1. Measure flour and cornmeal into a zip-top plastic bag, seal, and shake well to combine. Add squid, seal, and shake well to coat.

2. Place a large skillet over medium heat. Add enough olive oil to reach a depth of 2".

3. Loop some floured rings over the handle of a wooden spoon until you have a good batch for frying; add rings to oil one by one in a clockwise fashion until pan is full. Keep an eye on the time—at the 2½ minute mark remove rings in clockwise order from your starting point in the pan.

4. Place cooked calamari on a plate lined with paper towels to drain until all squid has been cooked. Repeat process with remaining calamari until all are cooked.

5. Sprinkle calamari with lemon juice and serve immediately.

PER SERVING Calories: 132 | Fat: 9.2 g | Protein: 5.4 g | Sodium: 12 mg | Fiber: 0.9 g | Carbohydrates: 7.2 g | Sugar: 0.2 g

Baked Tofu with Tangy Dipping Sauce

*Anything but bland, these breaded oven-fried cutlets will make a
tofu lover out of you! Paired with a sweet, slightly spicy sauce, they're
absolutely delicious. Double the quantity of tofu for larger parties.*

PREP TIME: 10 minutes
COOK TIME: 25 minutes

INGREDIENTS | SERVES 8

Olive oil cooking spray
1 pound extra-firm tofu, drained
1 large egg white
1 tablespoon water
½ cup bread crumbs
1 tablespoon dried parsley
1 teaspoon dried Italian seasoning
1 teaspoon ground paprika
1 teaspoon onion powder
½ teaspoon garlic powder
½ teaspoon freshly ground black pepper
1 (8-ounce) can tomato sauce
1 tablespoon apple cider vinegar
1 tablespoon molasses
1 tablespoon honey
1 tablespoon ground mustard
½ teaspoon ground cumin
⅛ teaspoon ground cayenne

Versatile Tofu

Tofu soaks up flavors like nothing else, and
can be added to almost any type of dish,
providing added protein, calcium, and iron.
Cube a pound of tofu, add to assorted
vegetables, and roast. Slice into sticks, toss
with a little nutritional yeast, and bake.
Crumble and add to a vegetable stir-fry
with brown rice. Or use instead of chicken
in a vegetarian noodle soup.

1. Preheat oven to 425°F. Spray a baking sheet lightly with cooking spray and set aside.

2. Gently press drained tofu between paper towels to release excess liquid. Slice tofu in half lengthwise, then slice each half into 8 equal pieces.

3. Beat egg white and water in a shallow bowl until slightly foamy.

4. Place bread crumbs in a medium bowl; add parsley, Italian seasoning, paprika, onion powder, garlic powder, and pepper and whisk well to combine.

5. Dip each piece of tofu in egg white, then press into the bread crumbs to coat. Place coated tofu cutlets on prepared baking sheet.

6. Place baking sheet on middle rack in oven and bake 10 minutes. Remove from oven, gently flip, and return to oven to bake another 10 minutes.

7. While tofu is baking, combine tomato sauce, vinegar, molasses, honey, mustard, cumin, and cayenne in a small saucepan. Heat over medium-low heat and stir frequently until mixture begins to bubble, about 3–5 minutes. Remove from heat and pour into a small serving bowl.

8. Remove tofu from oven and serve immediately with Tangy Dipping Sauce.

PER SERVING Calories: 123 | Fat: 4.0 g | Protein: 8.0 g | Sodium: 229 mg | Fiber: 2.0 g | Carbohydrates: 13.8 g | Sugar: 6.5 g

Glazed Balsamic Chicken Wings

Chicken wings are consummate party food. Here's a less guilty way of satisfying that indulgence. This recipe produces deliciously sticky wings with a crispy, caramelized coating that are truly finger-licking good!

PREP TIME: 10 minutes
COOK TIME: 35 minutes

INGREDIENTS | SERVES 6

3 pounds chicken wings, wing tips removed
½ cup red currant jelly
⅓ cup balsamic vinegar
1 teaspoon low-sodium soy sauce
1 teaspoon ground cayenne
1 teaspoon garlic powder
1 teaspoon onion powder

1. Preheat oven to 450°F. Line a baking sheet with aluminum foil and set aside.

2. Place wings in a large mixing bowl and set aside.

3. Measure jelly, vinegar, and soy sauce into a small saucepan. Place over medium-high heat and bring to a boil, stirring occasionally. Boil 5–7 minutes until mixture turns thick and glossy.

4. While mixture is boiling, measure cayenne, garlic powder, and onion powder into a small mixing bowl. Whisk well to combine.

5. Remove thickened jelly mixture from heat and whisk in seasoning mixture. Pour mixture over wings and toss well to coat.

6. Arrange coated wings on the baking sheet meaty-side down. Place baking sheet on middle rack in oven and bake 10–12 minutes. Flip wings, then return to oven and bake another 10–12 minutes.

7. Transfer remaining sauce in the bowl to a small saucepan, place over medium-high heat, and bring to a boil. Reduce heat to low and simmer 1–2 minutes.

8. At the end of the baking time, turn on the broiler and broil wings 3–4 minutes more until chicken is richly colored and glossy. Remove from oven and drizzle remaining sauce over wings. Serve immediately.

PER SERVING Calories: 267 | Fat: 4.5 g | Protein: 37.7 g | Sodium: 172 mg | Fiber: 0.3 g | Carbohydrates: 12.5 g | Sugar: 8.7 g

Lemony Herbed Chicken Wings

This recipe is flavored with a little olive oil, some rosemary, garlic, and the secret ingredient—lemon juice. This citrusy marinade imbues the chicken with moist flavor and the most delectable aroma. Allow the chicken to rest in the marinade as long as possible, preferably overnight.

PREP TIME: 8–12 hours
COOK TIME: 60 minutes

INGREDIENTS | SERVES 8

4 pounds chicken wings, wing tips removed
⅓ cup fresh or bottled lemon juice
⅓ cup olive oil
1 tablespoon dried rosemary, crushed
4 small cloves garlic, minced
½ teaspoon freshly ground black pepper

Waste Not, Want Not

Animal bones can't be composted, but they can be used to flavor recipes, especially homemade broth. Place bones and other scraps in a stockpot, add water to cover, and bring to a boil over high heat. Once boiling, reduce heat to low, cover, and simmer an hour or more. When it comes to vegetable trimmings, do the same. Peels, leaves, and stems may be unappealing to eat, but add a lot of flavor to stock. Save discarded scraps in plastic bags, seal, and freeze for later use.

1. Arrange chicken wings in an ovensafe baking dish without crowding; if necessary use two dishes. Set aside.

2. Measure remaining ingredients into a small mixing bowl and whisk well to combine. Pour over chicken wings and turn to coat.

3. Cover the dish and refrigerate as long as possible, preferably 8 hours or even overnight. Turn wings at least once while marinating.

4. When ready to cook, preheat oven to 400°F. Place wings in uncovered dish on middle rack in oven and bake until golden and crisp, 30–60 minutes depending upon the size of the wings. The internal temperature should reach 165°F and the juices should run clear. Remove from oven and let cool.

5. Serve warm or at room temperature. Wings can also be refrigerated for later consumption and served cold.

PER SERVING Calories: 278 | Fat: 11.0 g | Protein: 37.5 g | Sodium: 138 mg | Fiber: 0.3 g | Carbohydrates: 1.3 g | Sugar: 0.2 g

Roasted Chickpeas

Roasted chickpeas make an absolutely delicious snack, especially when they're eaten straight out of the oven. Serve them as a warm appetizer in a bowl, just as you would nuts, or toss them with salads instead of croutons. They're totally addictive, so watch out—you may find yourself eating more than just the ¼-cup serving!

PREP TIME: 5 minutes
COOK TIME: 30 minutes

INGREDIENTS | SERVES 8

1 teaspoon plus 1 tablespoon olive oil, divided

2 (15-ounce) cans chickpeas, drained, rinsed, and patted dry

1 teaspoon all-purpose seasoning

½ teaspoon freshly ground black pepper

1. Preheat oven to 400°F. Lightly oil a medium cast-iron skillet or baking sheet with 1 teaspoon olive oil and set aside.

2. Add remaining ingredients to a medium mixing bowl and toss well to coat.

3. Transfer chickpeas to the skillet or baking sheet and spread evenly. Place on middle rack in oven and bake 10 minutes. Stir chickpeas and bake another 10 minutes. Stir one more time and bake a final 10 minutes.

4. Remove from oven and serve immediately.

PER SERVING Calories: 105 | Fat: 3.0 g | Protein: 4.5 g | Sodium: 134 mg | Fiber: 4.0 g | Carbohydrates: 14.7 g | Sugar: 2.5 g

Curried Potato Croquettes

Samosas are absolutely delicious, but making them the traditional way with a fried pastry crust is not only time prohibitive but unhealthy. Fortunately, this recipe gives you faster, guilt-free samosas. Here the potato filling is rolled in bread crumbs, then oven baked. The resulting croquettes have a ton of flavor and a crisp outer crust, but are very low in fat. The recipe yields 24 croquettes, enough to serve 12 people as an appetizer or 8 as a main course. Serve with chutney or ketchup.

PREP TIME: 20 minutes
COOK TIME: 25 minutes

INGREDIENTS | SERVES 12

3 teaspoons olive oil, divided
6 medium potatoes, peeled and diced
2 tablespoons nutritional yeast
2 teaspoons ground cumin
2 teaspoons curry powder
1½ teaspoons garlic powder
1 teaspoon brown sugar
1 teaspoon cumin seeds
¾ teaspoon dried oregano
½ teaspoon ground coriander
¼ teaspoon ground cayenne
¼ teaspoon ground ginger
1 tablespoon low-sodium soy sauce
2 tablespoons chopped fresh cilantro
¾ cup bread crumbs

Preserving Dried Herbs and Spices

Many people position their spice rack close to the stove for easy access during cooking. But the proximity of the heat and humidity compromises flavor. To maximize freshness, store dried herbs and seasonings in a cool, dark cabinet away from direct sunlight and cooking.

1. Preheat oven to 400°F. Use 1 teaspoon olive oil to lightly oil two baking sheets and set aside.

2. Place potatoes in a medium stockpot and add enough water to cover by 1–2". Bring to a boil over high heat, then reduce heat to medium and boil 20 minutes.

3. While potatoes are cooking, add nutritional yeast, cumin powder, curry powder, garlic powder, sugar, cumin seeds, oregano, coriander, cayenne, and ginger to a small mixing bowl and whisk well to combine.

4. Drain potatoes, then mash. Add seasoning mixture, soy sauce, 2 teaspoons oil, and cilantro and stir to combine.

5. Place bread crumbs in a shallow bowl.

6. To form croquettes, scoop roughly 2 tablespoons potato mixture, roll into a ball, and flatten into a 2–3" patty. Press potato cake into bread crumbs, then gently flip to coat second side. Place breaded croquette on the baking sheet and repeat with remaining ingredients until you have 24 croquettes.

7. Place the baking sheets on the middle rack in the oven and bake 12–15 minutes until golden brown on the bottom. Gently flip, return to oven, and bake another 12–15 minutes until golden brown.

8. Remove from oven and serve immediately.

PER SERVING Calories: 114 | Fat: 1.5 g | Protein: 3.6 g | Sodium: 149 mg | Fiber: 2.0 g | Carbohydrates: 22.3 g | Sugar: 1.3 g

Sweet Clementine Salsa

As colorful as it is tangy, this bright orange salsa is bursting with citrus. Easy-peel clementines make preparation a snap; feel free to substitute another citrus fruit in the off-season. Pulse minimally in your food processor for an extra-chunky salsa to enjoy with chips, or purée for a fat-free drizzle to use over salads, grilled meat, and more.

PREP TIME: 5 minutes
COOK TIME: N/A

INGREDIENTS | YIELDS 1½ CUPS

4 small clementines, peeled

1 small red onion, peeled and quartered

2 cloves garlic

½ medium orange bell pepper, seeded and quartered

1 tablespoon fresh cilantro

1 tablespoon orange juice

1 teaspoon apple cider vinegar

¼ teaspoon ground cumin

⅛ teaspoon dried red pepper flakes

⅛ teaspoon chili seasoning

1. Place all ingredients in a food processor; cover and pulse to combine.

2. Cover and refrigerate until serving.

PER ¼-CUP SERVING Calories: 33 | Fat: 0.0 g | Protein: 0.8 g | Sodium: 3 mg | Fiber: 1.2 g | Carbohydrates: 8.3 g | Sugar: 5.2 g

Clementine Facts

Clementines are hugely popular, not only for their taste, but for their easy-to-peel skin. A cross between a Chinese mandarin and a conventional orange, they're slightly sweeter than an orange, but actually lower in sugar. Clementines are low in calories and high in vitamin C, potassium, beta carotene, and fiber, and they even contain calcium! Look for them beginning in the fall; their peak season stretches into the new year.

Green Pea Guacamole

Chunky, flavorful, and totally satisfying, this avocado-free dip has all the traditional taste without the fat. Bonus? Its gorgeous green color doesn't fade or turn brown, even after days in the refrigerator. Serve with chips or dollop over nachos, tacos, burritos, and more.

PREP TIME: 5 minutes
COOK TIME: 5 minutes

INGREDIENTS | YIELDS 2½ CUPS

2½ cups frozen peas

¼ cup water

1 small red onion, peeled and quartered

1 small fresh jalapeño pepper, seeded (if desired) and quartered

1 small ripe tomato, quartered

1 tablespoon fresh cilantro

1 small clove garlic

1 tablespoon lime juice

1 tablespoon olive oil

¼ teaspoon ground coriander

¼ teaspoon ground cumin

½ teaspoon freshly ground black pepper

1. Place peas and water in a microwave-safe bowl, cover with plastic wrap, and microwave 5 minutes on high. Drain and place in a food processor. Pulse to chop coarsely.

2. Add remaining ingredients to food processor; cover and pulse to combine.

3. Cover and refrigerate until serving.

PER ¼-CUP SERVING Calories: 48 | Fat: 1.4 g | Protein: 2.3 g | Sodium: 130 mg | Fiber: 2.5 g | Carbohydrates: 7.0 g | Sugar: 2.4 g

Basil Pesto Hummus

This absolutely scrumptious hummus is light and fluffy and flavored with the fresh taste of basil. It's also a nutritional powerhouse, high in vitamins (A, C, and K), folic acid, antioxidants, protein, and fiber. Partner with tortilla chips and fresh vegetables for a perfect party tray. Baby spinach may be substituted for the fresh arugula, if desired.

PREP TIME: 5 minutes
COOK TIME: N/A

INGREDIENTS | YIELDS 2 CUPS

¼ cup walnuts

⅓ cup fresh basil

⅓ cup fresh arugula

4 cloves garlic, minced

3 tablespoons nutritional yeast

1 tablespoon lemon juice

1 tablespoon low-sodium soy sauce

1 tablespoon olive oil

1 tablespoon tahini

½ teaspoon freshly ground black pepper

1 (15-ounce) can chickpeas, drained and liquid reserved

1. Place walnuts in a food processor and pulse until chopped.

2. Add basil, arugula, garlic, nutritional yeast, lemon juice, soy sauce, oil, tahini, pepper, chickpeas, and 4 tablespoons reserved chickpea liquid and pulse until smooth.

3. Serve immediately or cover and refrigerate until serving.

PER ¼-CUP SERVING Calories: 104 | Fat: 5.2 g | Protein: 4.5 g | Sodium: 136 mg | Fiber: 3.5 g | Carbohydrates: 10.5 g | Sugar: 1.5 g

Flavor Your Hummus

Instead of basil hummus, try something different. Make plain hummus by puréeing a 15-ounce can of chickpeas with 3 tablespoons tahini, 3 tablespoons lemon juice, 2 tablespoons olive oil, and 3 cloves garlic. Make it more citrusy by adding the grated zest of a fresh lemon. For a spicy Southwestern hummus, skip the lemon juice and add lime juice, minced jalapeño, ground cumin, and a little chili seasoning. Make a tasty Asian-style hummus using five-spice powder, ginger, low-sodium soy sauce, sesame oil, and scallions. Or create a vegetable-centric hummus by adding puréed sautéed vegetables and a little broth.

Crisp and Crunchy Kale Popcorn

If you like kale chips, you're going to love this yummy snack. The flavored popcorn and crackly kale come together in a crisp and crunchy marriage of tastes and textures. It's a deliciously healthy, fun, and filling way to satisfy your between-meal cravings.

PREP TIME: 10 minutes
COOK TIME: 23 minutes

INGREDIENTS | SERVES 10

8 cups chopped fresh kale leaves
2 tablespoons nutritional yeast, divided
1½ teaspoons garlic powder, divided
½ teaspoon low-sodium soy sauce
½ teaspoon olive oil
1 teaspoon sriracha
8 cups air-popped popcorn
½ teaspoon ground cumin
½ teaspoon ground paprika
¼ teaspoon dried oregano
¼ teaspoon dried thyme
⅛ teaspoon ground cayenne
Olive oil cooking spray

1. Preheat oven to 300°F. Line two baking sheets with parchment and set aside.

2. Place kale in a large mixing bowl.

3. Measure 1 tablespoon nutritional yeast, ½ teaspoon garlic powder, soy sauce, oil, and sriracha into a small bowl and stir well to combine. Drizzle mixture over kale and toss 1–2 minutes using your hands to coat.

4. Spread kale evenly on the two baking sheets so the pieces have space between them. Place on middle rack in oven and bake 10 minutes. Stir gently, then bake another 3 minutes until kale is dark and crisp. Remove from oven and set aside.

5. Place popcorn in a large mixing bowl. Add cumin, paprika, oregano, thyme, and cayenne to a small bowl and stir to combine. Spray popcorn lightly with cooking spray, sprinkle with seasoning mix, and toss well to coat. Spread popcorn evenly on a parchment-lined baking sheet. Place on middle rack in oven and bake 5 minutes until mixture is lightly toasted.

6. Remove popcorn from the oven and transfer to a large mixing bowl. Add kale chips and toss gently to combine. Divide mixture evenly between two parchment-lined baking sheets, return to middle rack in oven, and bake another 3–5 minutes until toasted.

7. Remove from oven and place on wire rack to cool. Serve warm or cool.

PER SERVING Calories: 38 | Fat: 0.6 g | Protein: 1.9 g | Sodium: 22 mg | Fiber: 1.7 g | Carbohydrates: 7.0 g | Sugar: 0.5 g

Cinnamon-Sweet Cracker Jack Popcorn

Don't be fooled by the simplicity of this recipe! The resulting popcorn tastes like homemade Cracker Jack, but with very little sugar and zero salt. It has the perfect hint of sugar and spice and couldn't be easier to make. If you're feeling extra hungry, add ¼ cup of unsalted roasted peanuts, double the batch, and dig in! It's a guilt-free sweet and crunchy snack you can enjoy anytime.

PREP TIME: 2 minutes
COOK TIME: 10 minutes

INGREDIENTS | SERVES 4

1 tablespoon sugar
⅛ teaspoon ground cinnamon
4 cups air-popped popcorn
Olive oil cooking spray

Healthy Homemade Gifts

The most thoughtful gifts are often those you make yourself. Packaging nuts and other snacks in tins or glass containers is a tasty way of showing you care. At holiday time, there's nothing sweeter than sharing a tray of healthy, homemade baked goods. And remember, seasonings and condiments are practical as well as delicious. Presented in a pretty jar or squeeze bottle, they're a gift that keeps on giving.

1. Preheat oven to 300°F. Line a baking sheet with parchment and set aside.

2. Measure sugar and cinnamon into a small bowl and whisk well to combine. Add popcorn to a large bowl and spray with oil, then add cinnamon-sugar and toss well to coat.

3. Spread popcorn evenly on the baking sheet. Lightly spray again with oil and sprinkle with any residual seasoning. Place pan on middle rack in oven and bake 4–5 minutes. Stir mix, rotate pan, and bake another 4–5 minutes, until lightly golden.

4. Remove from oven and place on wire rack to cool. Serve warm or cool.

PER SERVING Calories: 42 | Fat: 0.3 g | Protein: 1.0 g | Sodium: 0 mg | Fiber: 1.2 g | Carbohydrates: 9.4 g | Sugar: 3.2 g

Party Mix Popcorn

An addictively crunchy alternative to potato chips and other salty snacks, this deliciously seasoned party mix will make a MIND diet snack lover out of you. For variety, substitute 2 cups of pretzels or bite-sized shredded wheat cereal for an equal amount of the popcorn.

PREP TIME: 5 minutes
COOK TIME: 10 minutes

INGREDIENTS | SERVES 10

10 cups air-popped popcorn
1 cup unsalted peanuts
2 tablespoons nutritional yeast
1 tablespoon low-sodium soy sauce
1 teaspoon garlic powder
½ teaspoon onion powder
½ teaspoon lemon-pepper seasoning
¼ teaspoon dried dill
⅛ teaspoon ground mustard
Olive oil cooking spray

1. Preheat oven to 300°F. Line two baking sheets with parchment and set aside.

2. Place popcorn and peanuts in a large mixing bowl.

3. Measure nutritional yeast, soy sauce, garlic powder, onion powder, lemon-pepper, dill, and mustard into a small bowl and whisk well to combine. Spray popcorn mixture with oil, add seasoning blend, and toss well to coat; spray with a little more oil as necessary to get the seasoning to stick.

4. Spread party mix evenly on the prepared baking sheets. Lightly spray again with oil. Place pans on middle rack in oven and bake 4–5 minutes. Stir mix, rotate pans, and bake another 4–5 minutes, until lightly toasted.

5. Remove from oven and place on wire rack to cool. Serve warm or cool.

PER SERVING Calories: 122 | Fat: 6.7 g | Protein: 5.2 g | Sodium: 69 mg | Fiber: 2.6 g | Carbohydrates: 10.0 g | Sugar: 0.8 g

CHAPTER 8

Salads

Roasted Sweet Potato Salad with Kidney Beans and Peas

Roasted sweet potatoes drizzled with a spicy, sweet vinaigrette? What's not to love? Kidney beans, green peas, and chopped pecans add protein, color, and crunchy appeal, making this well-rounded salad one of the prettiest, tastiest, and healthiest yet! Substitute walnuts for the pecans if desired, and change the salad greens depending on the seasons: spring mix, arugula, baby spinach, or a blend of herbs and greens. For less spice, reduce the ground cayenne to ¼ teaspoon.

PREP TIME: 30 minutes
COOK TIME: 35 minutes

INGREDIENTS | SERVES 6

2 medium sweet potatoes, peeled and cut into 1" cubes

1 small onion, peeled and diced

2 teaspoons all-purpose seasoning

1 (15-ounce) can kidney beans, drained and rinsed

⅔ cup frozen peas, thawed

¼ cup chopped pecans

2 tablespoons apple juice

2 tablespoons apple cider vinegar

2 tablespoons olive oil

¼ cup chopped fresh parsley

1 teaspoon agave nectar

1 teaspoon chili seasoning

½ teaspoon ground cayenne

¼ teaspoon ground mustard

¼ teaspoon freshly ground black pepper

6 cups mixed salad greens

1. Preheat oven to 425°F. Line a baking sheet with parchment and set aside.

2. Place sweet potatoes in a large mixing bowl, add onion and all-purpose seasoning, and toss well. Spread in a single layer on the parchment, place baking sheet on middle rack in oven, and bake 35 minutes until tender.

3. Remove pan from oven and set aside.

4. Place kidney beans in a large bowl. Add peas, pecans, and sweet potatoes and toss gently to combine; set aside.

5. Add apple juice, vinegar, oil, parsley, agave, chili seasoning, cayenne, mustard, and pepper to a small mixing bowl and whisk well to combine. Pour dressing over sweet potatoes and toss gently to coat.

6. Plate greens and spoon sweet potato mixture over top. Serve warm or cold.

PER SERVING Calories: 159 | Fat: 7.8 g | Protein: 4.8 g | Sodium: 182 mg | Fiber: 5.4 g | Carbohydrates: 20.1 g | Sugar: 4.3 g

Chickpea Zucchini Salad

A toothsome combination of flavors and textures makes this salad a favorite in every season, but it's especially tasty in summer made with fresh garden zucchini. If you have fresh dill, substitute 1 teaspoon for the dried. Kelp granules are sold in many supermarkets and health-food stores; they add a distinctive, slightly fishy flavor. One bite of this salad and you'll be hooked!

PREP TIME: 10 minutes
COOK TIME: N/A

INGREDIENTS | SERVES 4

1 (15-ounce) can chickpeas, drained and rinsed

1 medium zucchini, diced

½ small onion, peeled and minced

2 tablespoons lemon juice

2 tablespoons olive oil

1 tablespoon nutritional yeast

½ teaspoon all-purpose seasoning

¼ teaspoon dried dill

¼ teaspoon dried herbes de Provence

¼ teaspoon kelp granules

1. Place chickpeas in a medium mixing bowl. Add zucchini and onion and toss gently to combine. Set aside.

2. Measure remaining ingredients into a small mixing bowl and whisk together. Pour dressing over salad and toss well to coat.

3. Cover and refrigerate until serving.

PER SERVING Calories: 164 | Fat: 7.8 g | Protein: 5.7 g | Sodium: 146 mg | Fiber: 4.9 g | Carbohydrates: 17.9 g | Sugar: 4.2 g

What Is Nutritional Yeast?

Nutritional yeast is a type of inactive yeast with a zingy, cheese-like flavor, making it a great substitute for cheese in the MIND diet. The little yellow flakes can be sprinkled on popcorn, pasta, or anything you'd like to perk up. Some nutritional yeast also contains important vitamins such as B_{12}, often found in meat, making it an especially nutritious supplement for vegetarians and vegans. Nutritional yeast is sold in health-food stores, the natural food section of some supermarkets, and online. To save time and money, buy it in bulk and store it in an airtight container in the freezer.

Asian Cucumber Salad

Tangy, crisp, and irresistible, this salad comes together in minutes and will be gone just as fast. Enjoy it immediately or cover and refrigerate; the flavors only improve with time. If you don't have the seedless variety, substitute 2 medium peeled and seeded conventional cucumbers instead. For added appeal use a red onion and sprinkle the salad with toasted sesame seeds before serving.

PREP TIME: 10 minutes
COOK TIME: N/A

INGREDIENTS | SERVES 4

1 large seedless cucumber, sliced diagonally into ¼" slices

1 small onion, peeled, halved, and sliced

1 clove garlic, minced

2 tablespoons natural (unflavored) rice wine vinegar

1 tablespoon olive oil

1 teaspoon sesame oil

1 teaspoon low-sodium soy sauce

1 teaspoon agave nectar

1 teaspoon all-purpose seasoning

¼ teaspoon ground ginger

⅛ teaspoon dried red pepper flakes

¼ teaspoon freshly ground black pepper

1. Place cucumber, onion, and garlic in a medium mixing bowl and mix well to combine. Set aside.

2. Measure remaining ingredients into a small mixing bowl and whisk well to combine. Pour dressing over salad and toss well to coat.

3. Cover and refrigerate until serving.

PER SERVING Calories: 60 | Fat: 4.4 g | Protein: 0.7 g | Sodium: 42 mg | Fiber: 0.8 g | Carbohydrates: 4.4 g | Sugar: 2.6 g

Vegetable Pasta Salad with Zesty Italian Dressing

*Perfect for potlucks, picnics, and barbecues, this pasta salad
will be the hit of the party. The recipe makes enough to
serve 12, half when feeding a smaller group. Make ahead
and refrigerate; the salad keeps well for several days.*

PREP TIME: 15 minutes
COOK TIME: 15 minutes

INGREDIENTS | SERVES 12

1 pound dry whole-grain rotini or similar pasta

1 medium red onion, peeled and diced

2 cups grape tomatoes

1 medium seedless cucumber, diced

1 medium red bell pepper, seeded and diced

3 cups chopped fresh broccoli

1 medium yellow squash, diced

1 medium zucchini, diced

1 (15-ounce) can chickpeas, drained and rinsed

⅓ cup olives, sliced

8 tablespoons olive oil

4 tablespoons apple cider vinegar

4 tablespoons white distilled vinegar

4 tablespoons water

3 tablespoons nutritional yeast

1½ teaspoons agave nectar

1½ teaspoons dried oregano

1 teaspoon all-purpose seasoning

1 teaspoon dried parsley

1 teaspoon garlic powder

1 teaspoon onion powder

¼ teaspoon dried basil

¼ teaspoon freshly ground black pepper

⅛ teaspoon dried thyme

1. Cook pasta according to directions. Drain and set aside.

2. Place onion, tomatoes, cucumber, bell pepper, broccoli, squash, zucchini, chickpeas, and olives in an extra-large mixing bowl. Add pasta. Set aside.

3. Measure remaining ingredients into a small mixing bowl and whisk well to combine. Pour dressing over salad and toss well to coat.

4. Serve salad immediately or cover and refrigerate until serving.

PER SERVING Calories: 278 | Fat: 10.6 g | Protein: 8.2 g | Sodium: 85 mg | Fiber: 7.4 g | Carbohydrates: 38.8 g | Sugar: 5.4 g

Low-Sodium Caesar Salad

This low-sodium version of the classic salad doesn't require any raw eggs (so there isn't a risk of salmonella) or any anchovies (so even the kids will love it). The dressing is a simple pulsed-together concoction of olive oil, lemon juice, and garlic, whisked with a combination of sour cream and shredded Swiss cheese, which is perfect when you decide to have your weekly taste of dairy. The tossed salad is sprinkled with a kiss of Parmesan and freshly ground pepper, resulting in an irresistibly tangy, creamy, crunchy, and delicious garlicky dish that you'll make over and over again.

PREP TIME: 5 minutes
COOK TIME: N/A

INGREDIENTS | SERVES 6

4 tablespoons olive oil

2 tablespoons lemon juice

4 cloves garlic

⅛ teaspoon ground white pepper

½ cup fat-free sour cream

½ cup shredded Swiss cheese

18 ounces or 9 cups chopped fresh romaine lettuce

1 tablespoon grated Parmesan cheese

¼ teaspoon freshly ground black pepper

1. Measure oil and lemon juice into a food processor. Add garlic and white pepper, then cover and pulse until smooth. Pour dressing into a small mixing bowl, add sour cream and Swiss cheese, and stir until combined.

2. Place romaine in a large salad bowl, spoon dressing over top, and toss gently to coat. Sprinkle with Parmesan and black pepper.

3. Serve immediately.

PER SERVING Calories: 147 | Fat: 11.5 g | Protein: 4.3 g | Sodium: 54 mg | Fiber: 1.6 g | Carbohydrates: 7.0 g | Sugar: 1.2 g

The Best 3-Bean Salad Ever!

Colorful, tangy, and ready in mere minutes, this protein-packed salad is sure to become a family favorite. Spoon this salad over mixed greens or use large lettuce leaves as "bowls" for fun.

PREP TIME: 5 minutes
COOK TIME: N/A

INGREDIENTS | SERVES 8

1 (15-ounce) can black beans, drained and rinsed

1 (15-ounce) can chickpeas, drained and rinsed

1 (15-ounce) can kidney beans, drained and rinsed

1 small onion, peeled and minced

3 medium stalks celery, trimmed and diced

1 small red bell pepper, seeded and diced

⅓ cup olive oil

⅓ cup apple cider vinegar

⅓ cup agave nectar

¼ teaspoon freshly ground black pepper

1. Place beans in a salad bowl. Add onion, celery, and bell pepper and stir to combine.

2. Measure remaining ingredients into a small mixing bowl and whisk well to combine. Pour dressing over salad and toss well to coat.

3. Serve immediately or cover and refrigerate until serving.

PER SERVING Calories: 332 | Fat: 9.8 g | Protein: 14.1 g | Sodium: 332 mg | Fiber: 14.4 g | Carbohydrates: 47.3 g | Sugar: 13.6 g

Marinated Mushroom Salad

This Marinated Mushroom Salad is absolutely amazing. Substitute an equal amount of roasted red pepper for the sun-dried tomatoes if you prefer. Serve over greens for a deliciously different salad, partner with hummus and unsalted chips as a fabulous dip, or use as a savory topping for pizza. For a spicier version, add ⅛–¼ teaspoon dried red pepper flakes to the dressing.

PREP TIME: 4–8 hours
COOK TIME: N/A

INGREDIENTS | SERVES 8

10 ounces fresh mushrooms, diced
1 small zucchini, diced
1 small yellow squash, diced
¼ cup chopped sun-dried tomatoes
4 tablespoons olive oil
2 tablespoons lemon juice
2 tablespoons apple cider vinegar
2 tablespoons nutritional yeast
1 teaspoon agave nectar
¾ teaspoon garlic powder
½ teaspoon all-purpose seasoning
½ teaspoon dried basil
½ teaspoon ground mustard
¼ teaspoon dried oregano
¼ teaspoon freshly ground black pepper

1. Place mushrooms, zucchini, squash, and tomatoes in a large bowl and stir to combine. Set aside.

2. Measure remaining ingredients into a small mixing bowl and whisk well to combine. Pour dressing over vegetables and stir well to coat.

3. Cover and refrigerate at least 4 hours, preferably overnight; stir occasionally.

PER SERVING Calories: 85 | Fat: 6.8 g | Protein: 2.3 g | Sodium: 9 mg | Fiber: 1.2 g | Carbohydrates: 4.7 g | Sugar: 2.8 g

Mandarin Chicken Salad with Spinach and Pecans

This healthy take on a perennial restaurant favorite gives you all the flavor of the traditional dish, but is perfect for the MIND diet. It makes the most of the canned fruit by incorporating the juice into the dressing; no added sugar is necessary. If you don't have red wine vinegar, substitute apple cider vinegar instead.

PREP TIME: 10 minutes
COOK TIME: N/A

INGREDIENTS | SERVES 4

1 (5-ounce) can mandarin oranges in juice, drained and liquid reserved

2 tablespoons olive oil

2 tablespoons red wine vinegar

1 tablespoon nutritional yeast

1 teaspoon agave nectar

1 teaspoon all-purpose seasoning

1 teaspoon stoneground mustard

⅛ teaspoon garlic powder

⅛ teaspoon freshly ground black pepper

1 small red onion, peeled and finely sliced

¼ cup dried cranberries

⅓ cup chopped pecans

2 (6-ounce) cooked boneless, skinless chicken breasts, diced

8 cups fresh baby spinach

1. Measure out 2 tablespoons mandarin juice and place in a small mixing bowl. Add oil, vinegar, nutritional yeast, agave, seasoning, mustard, garlic powder, and pepper. Whisk well to combine.

2. Place mandarin oranges, onion, cranberries, pecans, chicken, and spinach in a large salad bowl. Pour dressing over salad and toss well to coat.

3. Serve immediately.

PER SERVING Calories: 282 | Fat: 14.4 g | Protein: 21.8 g | Sodium: 51 mg | Fiber: 3.7 g | Carbohydrates: 16.6 g | Sugar: 10.4 g

Chicken Facts

Chicken's mild flavor and affordability make it one of the most popular proteins in the world. When preparing chicken, first remove the skin; this will greatly reduce the amount of fat you're consuming. White meat contains less fat, but dark meat contains a higher concentration of some nutrients. Skinless chicken is an excellent source of protein, vitamin B_6, and minerals such as iron.

Roasted Eggplant Salad with Walnuts

This salad is packed full of seductively soft, oven-roasted eggplant, red pepper, and caramelized onion, with a hint of fresh lemon and the bright bite of parsley and walnuts. Serve it over salad greens, partner with your choice of protein, or use as a delicious filling for vegetable sandwiches—and don't forget the hummus!

PREP TIME: 10 minutes
COOK TIME: 40 minutes

INGREDIENTS | SERVES 4

1 large eggplant, peeled and cut into 1" cubes

2 medium red bell peppers, seeded and diced

1 large onion, peeled and diced

2 tablespoons olive oil

2 tablespoons lemon juice

1 tablespoon nutritional yeast

2 teaspoons agave nectar

2 teaspoons low-sodium soy sauce

1 teaspoon all-purpose seasoning

1 teaspoon garlic powder

¼ teaspoon freshly ground black pepper

⅓ cup chopped walnuts

¼ cup chopped fresh parsley

1. Preheat oven to 400°F. Line a baking sheet with parchment and set aside.

2. Place eggplant, red peppers, and onion in a large mixing bowl. Add oil, lemon juice, nutritional yeast, agave, soy sauce, seasoning, garlic powder, and black pepper. Toss well to coat.

3. Spread mixture evenly onto the baking sheet. Place sheet on middle rack in oven and bake until tender, about 40 minutes.

4. Remove from oven and transfer to a large bowl. Add walnuts and parsley and toss well.

5. Serve immediately or cover and refrigerate until serving.

PER SERVING Calories: 197 | Fat: 12.9 g | Protein: 4.3 g | Sodium: 89 mg | Fiber: 6.0 g | Carbohydrates: 18.1 g | Sugar: 10.0 g

Sweet and Tangy Coleslaw with Jalapeño and Lime

This recipe gives run-of-the-mill coleslaw a modern kick! Celery seed, carrot, and mayonnaise are forsaken in favor of minced jalapeño, thinly sliced red bell pepper, and a citrus vinaigrette. It's a tantalizing twist on tradition, as pretty as it is tasty.

PREP TIME: 30–45 minutes
COOK TIME: 1½ minutes

INGREDIENTS | SERVES 6

4 tablespoons apple cider vinegar

2 tablespoons lime juice

2 tablespoons olive oil

¼ teaspoon freshly ground black pepper

6 cups shredded fresh cabbage

4 tablespoons sugar

1 large jalapeño pepper, seeded and minced

1 medium red bell pepper, seeded and diced

2 scallions, sliced

Jalapeño Facts

Jalapeños are a type of chili pepper native to Mexico. Used widely in many types of cuisine, the flavor and heat of the jalapeño melds well with many ingredients. To reduce the intensity of the jalapeño, remove its seeds and discard before adding to a dish; the flavor and some heat will remain. Jalapeños are high in fiber as well as vitamins C, B$_6$, and E, making them a healthy addition to any meal.

1. Measure vinegar, lime juice, oil, and black pepper into a large mixing bowl and whisk well to combine. Cover bowl and place in freezer to chill 15–30 minutes.

2. Place the cabbage in a microwave-safe bowl. Add sugar and toss to combine. Cover and microwave on high 1 minute. Remove, stir briefly, and re-cover. Microwave another 30 seconds or so until cabbage is slightly wilted and has reduced in volume by roughly a third. Carefully drain excess liquid.

3. Remove vinaigrette from freezer and add drained cabbage, along with jalapeño, bell pepper, and scallions; toss well to combine.

4. Cover and chill at least 15 minutes, then serve.

PER SERVING Calories: 98 | Fat: 4.4 g | Protein: 1.2 g | Sodium: 14 mg | Fiber: 2.3 g | Carbohydrates: 14.3 g | Sugar: 11.4 g

Salmon Salad with Whole-Wheat Couscous and Dill

This light, fluffy, and flavorful salad can be served warm or cold and even tastes great the next day. If you have fresh dill, by all means use it; add up to 2 tablespoons fresh chopped dill instead of the dried.

PREP TIME: 5 minutes
COOK TIME: 10 minutes

INGREDIENTS | SERVES 4

1¼ cup vegetable broth
1 cup uncooked whole-wheat couscous
2 tablespoons olive oil, divided
1 medium onion, peeled and chopped
2 cloves garlic, minced
⅔ cup frozen green peas
1 (8-ounce) can salmon, drained
3 tablespoons lemon juice
2 tablespoons nutritional yeast
2 teaspoons all-purpose seasoning
¾ teaspoon dried dill
¼ teaspoon freshly ground black pepper
6 cups fresh mixed salad greens

Speedy Salmon

When pressed for time, fresh or thawed frozen salmon can be prepared in mere minutes in the microwave. Wash the salmon and pat dry. Place the fillet in a microwave-safe dish and cover the top tightly with plastic wrap. Microwave for 3½ minutes. Check the thickest part for doneness; if any bright pink flesh is still showing, cover the dish again and return to the microwave for 30–45 seconds.

1. Measure broth into a 3-quart saucepan and bring to a boil over high heat. Add couscous, return to a simmer, then cover and remove from heat. Set aside 5 minutes.

2. Heat oil in a medium sauté pan over medium heat. Add onion and garlic and cook, stirring, 3 minutes. Add peas and cook, stirring, another 1–2 minutes. Remove pan from heat.

3. Fluff couscous and add to sauté pan. Flake salmon on top of the couscous. Sprinkle with lemon juice, nutritional yeast, seasoning, dill, and pepper. Toss gently to combine.

4. Serve immediately over greens or cover and refrigerate until serving.

PER SERVING Calories: 343 | Fat: 9.3 g | Protein: 23.6 g | Sodium: 646 mg | Fiber: 7.0 g | Carbohydrates: 47.2 g | Sugar: 4.0 g

Low-Sodium Greek Salad

This updated Greek salad is perfect for the MIND diet and retains much of the classic taste. Here, a tiny bit of feta enhances the flavor without a huge amount of salt, and the chickpeas add protein and heft. The parsley adds a bright burst of flavor, but if you don't have the fresh herb, feel free to omit.

PREP TIME: 15 minutes
COOK TIME: N/A

INGREDIENTS | SERVES 4

6 cups chopped fresh romaine lettuce

2 medium cucumbers, peeled, halved, seeded, and roughly chopped

3 ripe medium tomatoes, cut into wedges

1 medium bell pepper, seeded and diced

1 medium red onion, peeled and thinly sliced

1 (15-ounce) can chickpeas, drained and rinsed

¼ cup sliced olives

2 tablespoons feta cheese

¼ cup chopped fresh parsley

2 tablespoons olive oil

2 tablespoons red wine vinegar

2 tablespoons nutritional yeast

1½ teaspoons water

1½ teaspoons lemon juice

½ teaspoon agave nectar

½ teaspoon all-purpose seasoning

½ teaspoon dried oregano

⅛ teaspoon garlic powder

⅛ teaspoon freshly ground black pepper

1. Place romaine in a large salad bowl. Add cucumbers, tomatoes, bell pepper, onion, chickpeas, olives, feta, and parsley.

2. Measure remaining ingredients into a small mixing bowl and whisk well to combine. Pour dressing over salad and toss well to coat.

3. Serve immediately.

PER SERVING Calories: 237 | Fat: 9.8 g | Protein: 9.1 g | Sodium: 257 mg | Fiber: 9.0 g | Carbohydrates: 28.7 g | Sugar: 9.9 g

Parsley Facts

Parsley is an easy-growing herb that comes in two varieties, flat-leaf and curly, and has an amazing, distinctive flavor when eaten raw. Use it to add a refreshing taste and color to salads, dressings, and pastas. Parsley contains high levels of vitamins A, C, and K, as well as antioxidants, and may help prevent cardiovascular disease.

Garlicky Kale Salad

If you love garlic, then this is the salad for you. Here, the kale is coated and massaged with a tangy dressing that you'll find absolutely irresistible. The key to this amazing salad lies in preparing the kale. Trim the leaves, removing all fibrous stems, and tear into tiny pieces. Work the chopped kale with your hands for a couple of minutes before adding the dressing; after dressing, toss the salad vigorously with tongs for 3–5 minutes. All the handling softens the leaves and allows the flavors to fully permeate the salad.

PREP TIME: 10 minutes
COOK TIME: N/A

INGREDIENTS | SERVES 6

1 pound fresh kale, stems removed, leaves chopped (about 8 cups)
3 cloves garlic, minced
1 tablespoon olive oil
1 tablespoon tahini
1 tablespoon apple cider vinegar
1 tablespoon lemon juice
1 tablespoon low-sodium soy sauce
2 tablespoons nutritional yeast
¼ teaspoon freshly ground black pepper

1. Place kale in a large salad bowl and massage with your hands for a couple of minutes to soften.

2. Measure remaining ingredients into a small mixing bowl and whisk well to combine. Pour dressing over salad and toss to coat completely; work dressing into salad with tongs 3–5 minutes.

3. Serve immediately or cover and chill before serving. The salad may be made several hours ahead of serving; the longer it chills, the stronger the flavors.

PER SERVING Calories: 54 | Fat: 3.6 g | Protein: 2.3 g | Sodium: 98 mg | Fiber: 1.3 g | Carbohydrates: 3.7 g | Sugar: 0.6 g

What Is Tahini?

Tahini is a smooth paste made from ground sesame seeds. Its distinctive flavor is used to enhance many Middle Eastern dishes, including hummus, baba ghanoush, and halva. Tahini is sold in the international section of most supermarkets, and once opened it should be refrigerated to prevent spoilage.

Tuna Salad with White Beans and Tomatoes

Not only is this salad beautiful, but its incredible range of flavors is so impressive it'll make a salad fan of almost anyone! An equal amount of another cooked seafood, such as salmon or shrimp, may be substituted for the canned tuna if desired.

PREP TIME: 1 hour 15 minutes
COOK TIME: N/A

INGREDIENTS | SERVES 8

1 (15-ounce) can cannellini beans, drained and rinsed

1 (6-ounce) can tuna, drained

1 medium bell pepper, seeded and diced

1 small red onion, peeled and diced

2 medium stalks celery, trimmed and diced

1 large tomato, diced

2 scallions, thinly sliced

1 tablespoon chopped olives

2 tablespoons olive oil

2 tablespoons apple cider vinegar

2 tablespoons lemon juice

1 tablespoon tomato sauce

1 tablespoon nutritional yeast

1 teaspoon agave nectar

1 teaspoon all-purpose seasoning

½ teaspoon garlic powder

½ teaspoon dried oregano

½ teaspoon ground mustard

¼ teaspoon freshly ground black pepper

1. Place beans, tuna, bell pepper, onion, celery, tomato, scallions, and olives in a large salad bowl and toss gently.

2. Measure remaining ingredients into a small mixing bowl and whisk well to combine. Pour dressing over salad and toss well to coat.

3. Salad tastes best when allowed to marinate, so cover and refrigerate at least 1 hour, then serve.

PER SERVING Calories: 149 | Fat: 5.8 g | Protein: 9.8 g | Sodium: 100 mg | Fiber: 4.0 g | Carbohydrates: 14.6 g | Sugar: 2.5 g

Choose Canned Tuna Wisely

Studies show that many canned tunas exceed the FDA's advisory limits for mercury and should not be eaten often. When buying tuna, opt for chunk light over white albacore, as it is lower in mercury. Some brands, such as Oregon's Choice and Wild Planet, contain far lower levels of mercury and higher values of healthy omega-3 fatty acids.

Georgian Bean Salad with Caramelized Onions

This salad looks a little messy on the plate, but what it lacks in looks, it more than makes up for in taste. Toasted walnuts, caramelized onion, fresh herbs, and a splash of hot sauce embrace the heart of this salad: kidney beans. It's healthy, protein-rich, fiber-full, and absolutely delicious. For added vitamins and nutrients, stir in 5 ounces of fresh baby spinach at the end of cooking and allow it to wilt before serving.

PREP TIME: 10 minutes
COOK TIME: 10 minutes

INGREDIENTS | SERVES 6

½ cup chopped walnuts

2 tablespoons olive oil

1 large onion, peeled and thinly sliced

3 cloves garlic, minced

2 (15-ounce) cans kidney beans, drained and rinsed

¼ cup vegetable broth

1 tablespoon apple cider vinegar

1 tablespoon lemon juice

¼ cup chopped fresh cilantro

¼ cup chopped fresh parsley

1½ tablespoons nutritional yeast

1 teaspoon hot sauce

¼ teaspoon freshly ground black pepper

1. Heat a large sauté pan over medium heat. Add walnuts and toast, stirring, 2–3 minutes, until fragrant. Remove from pan and set aside. Wipe pan clean with a paper towel.

2. Add oil to pan and heat over medium heat. Add onion and cook, stirring, 4 minutes. Add garlic and cook, stirring, 30 seconds. Add beans and stir well to combine, 30 seconds.

3. Add broth, vinegar, and lemon juice and cook until the liquid has evaporated, stirring and scraping the residue from the bottom of the pan, 2–3 minutes.

4. Remove pan from heat. Add walnuts, cilantro, and parsley. Sprinkle with nutritional yeast, hot sauce, and pepper and stir well to combine.

5. Serve immediately.

PER SERVING Calories: 238 | Fat: 11.3 g | Protein: 10.8 g | Sodium: 258 mg | Fiber: 8.9 g | Carbohydrates: 24.6 g | Sugar: 0.4 g

Warm Potato Salad with Spinach

This salad shines with a light and flavorful vinaigrette. For added protein, toss in a handful of sunflower seeds or chopped walnuts, or expand the salad into a one-dish meal by adding thinly sliced red onion, fresh green beans, and cooked barley. Fingerlings may be substituted for the new potatoes.

PREP TIME: 10 minutes
COOK TIME: 15 minutes

INGREDIENTS | SERVES 8

3 pounds small new potatoes
4 cups fresh baby spinach
5 tablespoons red wine vinegar
5 tablespoons olive oil
2 tablespoons water
1 tablespoon mustard
1 tablespoon agave nectar
1 teaspoon garlic powder
1 teaspoon all-purpose seasoning
½ teaspoon dried dill
½ teaspoon dried Italian seasoning
½ teaspoon dried thyme
½ teaspoon freshly ground black pepper

1. Place unpeeled potatoes in a large pot and add enough water to cover by a couple of inches. Bring to a boil over high heat, then reduce heat to medium-high and simmer until tender, about 15 minutes.

2. Remove pot from heat and drain. Cut potatoes into bite-sized chunks.

3. Place potatoes back into the pot and add spinach.

4. In a small mixing bowl, whisk together remaining ingredients, then pour over potatoes and spinach. Toss well to coat and combine.

5. Serve immediately or cover and refrigerate until serving.

PER SERVING Calories: 221 | Fat: 8.5 g | Protein: 4.1 g | Sodium: 44 mg | Fiber: 4.4 g | Carbohydrates: 33.0 g | Sugar: 3.3 g

What Is Agave Nectar?

Agave nectar is a liquid sweetener derived from the agave cactus. It's a clear, light brown liquid, similar in appearance to maple syrup, though slightly thicker. It has a subtle, pleasant flavor and is very sweet, about twice as sweet as cane sugar. Because of its liquid form, it dissolves instantly, which makes it a great choice for sweetening beverages and dressings. Unlike honey, agave nectar is considered a vegan food.

Kale Salad with Pecan Parmesan and Dried Cranberries

If you don't make this salad, you'll never know how truly exquisite kale can be. The greens are dressed in a lemony lip-smacking vinaigrette, so good it'll make you lick your fork, then topped with dried sweetened cranberries and a tasty toasted pecan crumb. The combination of flavors is out of this world.

PREP TIME: 20 minutes
COOK TIME: 8 minutes

INGREDIENTS | SERVES 6

½ cup pecans

3 tablespoons nutritional yeast, divided

2½ tablespoons olive oil, divided

¾ teaspoon all-purpose seasoning, divided

½ teaspoon low-sodium soy sauce

1 pound fresh kale, stems removed, leaves finely chopped (roughly 8 cups)

3 cloves garlic, minced

4 tablespoons lemon juice

1 tablespoon agave nectar

¼ teaspoon freshly ground black pepper

½ cup dried sweetened cranberries

1. Preheat oven to 300°F. Spread pecans in a single layer on a baking sheet. Place sheet on middle rack in oven and bake 8 minutes until lightly toasted.

2. Transfer pecans to a food processor and chop until pea size. Add 1 tablespoon nutritional yeast, 1½ teaspoons oil, ¼ teaspoon all-purpose seasoning, and soy sauce; pulse into a coarse crumb. Set aside.

3. Place kale in a large salad bowl and set aside.

4. Measure garlic, lemon juice, remaining 2 tablespoons oil, remaining 2 tablespoons nutritional yeast, agave, remaining ½ teaspoon all-purpose seasoning, and pepper into a small food processor. Pulse until combined.

5. Pour dressing over kale and toss well to coat using tongs, 2 minutes. Top with pecan mixture and dried cranberries.

6. Serve immediately or cover and refrigerate before serving.

PER SERVING Calories: 170 | Fat: 11.4 g | Protein: 2.9 g | Sodium: 24 mg | Fiber: 2.8 g | Carbohydrates: 16.0 g | Sugar: 10.2 g

CHAPTER 9

Soups, Stews, and Chilies

Slow Cooker Lentil-Vegetable Soup

This tomato-rich, thick, and delicious soup isn't just healthy and satisfying. Thanks to the slow cooker, it's also convenient, making it that much easier to stay true to your diet. For ease, the recipe calls for fresh baby spinach; substitute an equal amount of standard fresh chopped spinach or frozen spinach if you prefer.

PREP TIME: 10 minutes
COOK TIME: 4–8 hours

INGREDIENTS | SERVES 8

1 large onion, peeled and diced

3 medium carrots, peeled and diced

2 medium stalks celery, trimmed and diced

3 cloves garlic, minced

1 cup dried lentils, rinsed

1 cup fresh or frozen corn

10 ounces fresh baby spinach

1 (15-ounce) can no salt added diced tomatoes, with juice

3 cups vegetable broth

3 cups vegetable juice

2 cups water

1 tablespoon low-sodium soy sauce

1 teaspoon all-purpose seasoning

1 teaspoon dried basil

½ teaspoon dried thyme

½ teaspoon freshly ground black pepper

1. Place all ingredients in a slow cooker and stir well to combine. It may be a bit crowded initially because of the spinach, but will quickly cook down.

2. Cover the slow cooker and cook on low 6–8 hours or on high 4–5 hours, stirring occasionally if possible. Cook until vegetables and lentils are tender. Serve hot.

PER SERVING Calories: 145 | Fat: 0.5 g | Protein: 8.6 g | Sodium: 493 mg | Fiber: 5.9 g | Carbohydrates: 28.9 g | Sugar: 5.7 g

Slow Cooker Southwestern Soup

This recipe gives you the seductively earthly flavors of the Southwest in a delicious vegetable soup. For a spicier version, add a minced jalapeño pepper or ¼–½ teaspoon ground cayenne at the start. Kidney beans may be substituted for the black beans if desired. If you don't care for quinoa, add ½ cup cooked chickpeas instead.

PREP TIME: 15 minutes
COOK TIME: 5–6 hours

INGREDIENTS | SERVES 8

1 medium onion, peeled and diced

3 medium carrots, peeled and

3 medium stalks celery, trimmed and diced

3 cloves garlic, minced

1 large sweet potato, peeled and diced

1 medium red bell pepper, seeded and diced

1 large tomato, diced

½ cup frozen corn

¼ cup dry quinoa, rinsed

1 (15-ounce) can black beans, drained and rinsed

6½ cups vegetable broth

2 tablespoons tomato paste

2 bay leaves

2 teaspoons ground cumin

1½ teaspoons agave nectar

1½ teaspoons apple cider vinegar

1 teaspoon dried oregano

1 teaspoon ground paprika

1 teaspoon chili seasoning

½ teaspoon dried thyme

½ teaspoon ground coriander

½ teaspoon freshly ground black pepper

1. Place all ingredients in a slow cooker and stir well to combine. Set to high, cover, and cook 5–6 hours, stirring occasionally if possible.

2. Serve hot.

PER SERVING Calories: 140 | Fat: 0.7 g | Protein: 6.7 g | Sodium: 924 mg | Fiber: 7.5 g | Carbohydrates: 28.2 g | Sugar: 7.8 g

Vegetable Pot Pie Stew

This crustless pot pie is the perfect go-to comfort meal. It is simple, inexpensive, and absolutely delicious. A traditional combination of vegetables simmered in a creamy, herb-flavored broth, it's best served over cooked brown rice or eggless noodles, or partnered with toasted bread or biscuits.

PREP TIME: 10 minutes
COOK TIME: 30 minutes

INGREDIENTS | SERVES 8

1 cup unsweetened plain almond milk

3 tablespoons white whole-wheat flour

2 cups vegetable broth

3 tablespoons nutritional yeast

1 tablespoon low-sodium soy sauce

2 teaspoons all-purpose seasoning

½ teaspoon dried thyme

½ teaspoon ground mustard

½ teaspoon ground sage

¼ teaspoon dried dill

1 teaspoon olive oil

1 medium onion, peeled and diced

4 cloves garlic, minced

3 medium carrots, peeled and diced

3 medium stalks celery, trimmed and diced

2 cups diced mushrooms

1 cup frozen peas

1 cup frozen corn

1 cup fresh or frozen green beans, cut into 1" pieces

1 pound red potatoes, diced

2 cups chopped fresh baby spinach

1 (15-ounce) can chickpeas, drained and rinsed

½ teaspoon freshly ground black pepper

1. Measure milk and flour into a medium mixing bowl and whisk until smooth. Add broth, nutritional yeast, soy sauce, seasoning, thyme, mustard, sage, and dill and whisk well until combined; set aside.

2. Heat oil in a large stockpot over medium heat. Add onion and cook, stirring, 2 minutes, until it begins to sweat. Add garlic, carrots, celery, and mushrooms and sauté 5 minutes, until mushrooms begin to release their juice.

3. Add peas, corn, green beans, potatoes, spinach, and chickpeas and stir to combine. Pour liquid over vegetables and stir to coat. Bring mixture to a boil over high heat, then lower heat, cover, and simmer until vegetables are tender, about 20 minutes.

4. Remove from heat. Season with pepper. Serve hot.

PER SERVING Calories: 173 | Fat: 1.9 g | Protein: 7.9 g | Sodium: 498 mg | Fiber: 7.3 g | Carbohydrates: 33.1 g | Sugar: 6.3 g

Slow Cooker Sweet Potato and Kale Stew

Think of this recipe as a one-way ticket to health. Chock-full of the good stuff—vitamins, antioxidants, iron, calcium, fiber, and more—and with the most stupendous combination of flavors, this hearty, MIND diet–approved stew will leave you feeling fantastic. Serve over cooked brown rice for a nutritionally complete meal.

PREP TIME: 15 minutes
COOK TIME: 6 hours

INGREDIENTS | SERVES 8

3 medium sweet potatoes, peeled and cubed

1 large onion, peeled and diced

3 medium carrots, peeled and sliced

5 cloves garlic, minced

1 medium red bell pepper, seeded and diced

8 cups chopped fresh kale leaves

1 (15-ounce) can no salt added diced tomatoes, with juice

1 (15-ounce) can kidney beans, drained and rinsed

4 cups vegetable broth

1 (15-ounce) can light coconut milk

2 tablespoons tomato paste

1 tablespoon agave nectar

1 tablespoon apple cider vinegar

1 tablespoon lime juice

1 tablespoon Thai red curry paste

1 tablespoon ground cumin

1 teaspoon ground paprika

1½ teaspoons all-purpose seasoning

1 teaspoon ground coriander

½ teaspoon dried oregano

¼ teaspoon dried thyme

½ teaspoon freshly ground black pepper

1. Place all ingredients in a slow cooker and carefully stir to combine (it will be quite full). Cover the slow cooker, set to high, and cook 6 hours, stirring occasionally if possible.

2. Serve hot.

PER SERVING Calories: 257 | Fat: 3.7 g | Protein: 7.4 g | Sodium: 768 mg | Fiber: 10.2 g | Carbohydrates: 49.9 g | Sugar: 12.9 g

Pumpkin-Ginger Soup

This Pumpkin-Ginger Soup is a vibrant and flavorful dish whose subtle sweetness adds sophistication to any meal, especially holiday celebrations. If you don't have fresh ginger, substitute ¾ teaspoon ground ginger. If fresh cubed pumpkin is available, use 2 cups instead of the canned purée.

PREP TIME: 10 minutes
COOK TIME: 30 minutes

INGREDIENTS | SERVES 4

1 tablespoon olive oil
1 medium onion, peeled and chopped
1 large stalk celery, trimmed and diced
4 medium carrots, peeled and diced
1 (15-ounce) can pumpkin purée
3 tablespoons minced fresh ginger
4 cups vegetable broth
1 tablespoon agave nectar
1 tablespoon apple cider vinegar
2 bay leaves
½ teaspoon ground cinnamon
¼ teaspoon dried oregano
¼ teaspoon dried thyme
⅛ teaspoon dried allspice
½ teaspoon freshly ground black pepper

1. Heat oil in a small stockpot over medium heat. Add onion and celery and sauté 3 minutes, until they begin to sweat. Add carrots and cook, stirring, 2 minutes, until they begin to sweat.

2. Add remaining ingredients and stir well to combine. Bring to a boil over high heat; then reduce heat to low, cover, and simmer 25 minutes, stirring occasionally.

3. Remove from heat. Remove bay leaves and discard. Use an immersion blender to purée the soup or transfer soup to a food processor and pulse until smooth.

4. Serve warm.

PER SERVING Calories: 119 | Fat: 3.7 g | Protein: 2.1 g | Sodium: 998 mg | Fiber: 5.6 g | Carbohydrates: 21.6 g | Sugar: 12.0 g

Pumpkin Facts

Pumpkins are a type of winter squash with a hard outer shell and firm inner flesh. Like all winter squash, pumpkins must be cooked before eating. To prepare a pie pumpkin, simply cut in half, remove the seeds, and place halves in a microwave-safe bowl. Add an inch or two of water and microwave on high roughly 20 minutes. Scoop out cooked purée and use as desired, or freeze for later use. Pumpkin is an excellent source of vitamins A and C and fiber.

Hearty Slow Cooker Black Bean Soup

This recipe gives you a slow-cooked soup that will fill your house with the most spectacular aroma! If you'd prefer to cook the soup on the stove, simply sauté the vegetables first in a tablespoon of olive oil, then add the remaining ingredients; bring to a boil, reduce heat, cover, and simmer 45–60 minutes to really bring out the flavors. For less spice, seed the jalapeño before mincing. And remember: don't drain the beans! The liquid becomes part of the stock.

PREP TIME: 10 minutes
COOK TIME: 5–7 hours

INGREDIENTS | SERVES 6

1 medium onion, peeled and diced

3 garlic cloves

2 medium stalks celery, trimmed and diced

1 medium green bell pepper, seeded and diced

1 medium red bell pepper, seeded and diced

1 jalapeño pepper, seeded and minced

1 (15-ounce) can no salt added diced tomatoes, with juice

3 (15-ounce) cans black beans, undrained

5 cups vegetable broth

⅓ cup red wine

1 tablespoon apple cider vinegar

1 tablespoon agave nectar

1 bay leaf

1 tablespoon ground cumin

2 teaspoons all-purpose seasoning

2 teaspoons ground paprika

1½ teaspoons dried oregano

1 teaspoon ground coriander

½ teaspoon dried thyme

¼ teaspoon dried red pepper flakes

½ teaspoon freshly ground black pepper

1. Place all ingredients in a slow cooker and stir well to combine. Cover, set to low, and cook 7 hours, or set to high and cook 5 hours, stirring occasionally if possible.

2. Before serving, transfer roughly a third of the soup to a food processor and purée. Return soup to slow cooker and stir to combine.

3. Serve hot.

PER SERVING Calories: 266 | Fat: 0.5 g | Protein: 16.7 g | Sodium: 1,101 mg | Fiber: 18.3 g | Carbohydrates: 48.2 g | Sugar: 12.2 g

Simple 1-Can Tomato Soup

This Simple 1-Can Tomato Soup is so ridiculously easy and delicious, you can make and enjoy it anytime. Partner this recipe with a nice toasted sandwich for a lovely lunch or light dinner.

PREP TIME: 5 minutes
COOK TIME: 22 minutes

INGREDIENTS | SERVES 4

1 tablespoon olive oil

1 medium onion, peeled and chopped

1 tablespoon tomato paste

3 cloves garlic, minced

2 teaspoons agave nectar

1 (15-ounce) can no salt added diced tomatoes, with juice

4 cups vegetable broth

3 tablespoons nutritional yeast

1 tablespoon balsamic vinegar

2 teaspoons ground paprika

½ teaspoon dried oregano

½ teaspoon dried thyme

½ teaspoon freshly ground black pepper

1. Heat oil in a large saucepan over medium heat. Add onion and cook, stirring, 5 minutes, until softened. Add tomato paste, garlic, and agave and cook, stirring, 1–2 minutes until paste darkens.

2. Add diced tomatoes, broth, nutritional yeast, vinegar, paprika, oregano, thyme, and pepper and stir to combine. Cover, bring soup to a boil over high heat, then reduce heat to medium-low and simmer covered 15 minutes.

3. Remove from heat and use an immersion blender to purée, or transfer soup to a food processor and pulse until smooth. Serve immediately.

PER SERVING Calories: 107 | Fat: 3.6 g | Protein: 3.2 g | Sodium: 1,020 mg | Fiber: 3.7 g | Carbohydrates: 17.2 g | Sugar: 10.2 g

Slow Cooker Minestrone Soup

The ingredients in this soup are fresh and seasonal. In the summer when garden produce is plentiful, swap the green beans for 2 small zucchini, yellow squash, or one of each. Either fresh or frozen green beans work well in this recipe. To stretch the soup further, feel free to add a cup of frozen corn and an extra cup of broth. For the pasta, use tiny shells or something similar.

PREP TIME: 10 minutes
COOK TIME: 5–6 hours

INGREDIENTS | SERVES 6

1 medium onion, peeled and diced

3 medium carrots, peeled and sliced

3 medium stalks celery, trimmed and sliced

3 cloves garlic, minced

2 cups green beans, cut into 1" pieces

2 (15-ounce) cans no salt added diced tomatoes, with juice

1 (15-ounce) can chickpeas, drained and rinsed

4 cups vegetable broth

1 bay leaf

2 tablespoons nutritional yeast

2 teaspoons all-purpose seasoning

½ teaspoon dried basil

½ teaspoon dried marjoram

½ teaspoon freshly ground black pepper

⅓ cup small uncooked whole-grain shells

1. Place all ingredients except pasta in a slow cooker and stir well to combine. Cover and cook on high 5 hours.

2. After 5 hours of cooking time, add pasta, stir to combine, and cover. Cook for 45 minutes before serving.

3. Serve hot.

PER SERVING Calories: 147 | Fat: 1.0 g | Protein: 6.7 g | Sodium: 814 mg | Fiber: 8.3 g | Carbohydrates: 29.5 g | Sugar: 10.0 g

Cheesy Potato Chowder

This creamy concoction of potatoes, chicken broth, and cheese will make even the staunchest critic a huge fan. If the potatoes are thin-skinned, leave the peel on for added nutrients and fiber. Be sure to dice the potatoes small to speed cooking time. White wine adds a lot of flavor, but if you avoid alcohol, substitute an equal amount of broth or a tablespoon or two of rice wine vinegar or white wine vinegar. For a vegetarian soup, use vegetable broth instead.

PREP TIME: 10 minutes
COOK TIME: 25 minutes

INGREDIENTS | SERVES 6

1 tablespoon olive oil

1 large onion, peeled and diced

3 medium stalks celery, trimmed and diced

2 cloves garlic, minced

7 medium potatoes, peeled and diced

4 cups chicken broth

⅓ cup dry white wine

½ teaspoon dried thyme

¼ teaspoon ground rosemary

⅛ teaspoon dried basil

½ teaspoon freshly ground black pepper

1 cup shredded Swiss cheese

1. Heat oil in a medium stockpot over medium heat. Add onion, celery, and garlic and sauté 5 minutes, until softened.

2. Add potato, broth, white wine, thyme, rosemary, basil, and pepper.

3. Bring to a boil over high heat; then reduce heat to low, cover, and simmer 20 minutes, until potatoes are tender.

4. Remove pot from heat. Transfer half of the soup to a food processor and pulse until smooth. Return soup to pot and stir well to combine.

5. Add cheese and stir until melted. Serve immediately.

PER SERVING Calories: 296 | Fat: 7.1 g | Protein: 11.1 g | Sodium: 656 mg | Fiber: 3.7 g | Carbohydrates: 45.0 g | Sugar: 3.7 g

Slow Cooker Mushroom, Bean, and Barley Soup

This slow-simmered version of the classic soup retains all the heft and hearty flavor of the original. The dried porcini mushrooms add tremendous depth, smoky taste, and meaty bite! If you don't have dried mushrooms, substitute 1¾ cups chopped fresh mushrooms instead. The dried multibean mix used in the soup is sold alongside other dried beans in the supermarket and is often labeled "16 bean soup." Discard the seasoning packet that accompanies the beans; it's full of additives.

PREP TIME: 10 minutes
COOK TIME: 8 hours

INGREDIENTS | SERVES 6

1 cup dried multibean mix, rinsed well

6 cups vegetable broth

1 (15-ounce) can no salt added diced tomatoes, with juice

1 small onion, peeled and diced

3 cloves garlic, minced

2 medium carrots, peeled and diced

2 medium stalks celery, trimmed and diced

½ cup uncooked pearl barley

½ ounce dried porcini mushrooms

1 bay leaf

2 teaspoons dried Italian seasoning

½ teaspoon freshly ground black pepper

6 cups chopped fresh baby spinach

1 tablespoon balsamic vinegar

1. Place beans, broth, tomatoes, onion, garlic, carrots, celery, barley, mushrooms, bay leaf, Italian seasoning, and pepper in a slow cooker; stir to combine. Cover, set to low, and cook 8 hours, stirring occasionally if possible.

2. Before serving, add spinach and vinegar and stir to combine. Cook until spinach wilts, about 15 minutes, then remove bay leaf and serve.

PER SERVING Calories: 250 | Fat: 1.0 g | Protein: 12.5 g | Sodium: 1,022 mg | Fiber: 13.7 g | Carbohydrates: 50.0 g | Sugar: 7.8 g

What Is Barley?

Barley is a type of whole grain, with a chewy texture and slightly nutty taste. Standard pearl barley cooks in about 40 minutes; quick barley is parboiled, allowing it to cook in a quarter of the time. Most of the barley grown in the United States is destined for beverages rather than food. Fermented barley, also known as barley malt, is an important ingredient in beer making. Barley is cholesterol-free, low in fat, and high in fiber.

Manhattan Seafood Stew

This intoxicating tomato-based stew is filled with an earthy richness (carrots, potatoes, onions, and garlic), the scent of the sea (fish and shrimp), a touch of citrus (orange zest), and a spicy kick (cilantro and spicy hot pepper). One bite and you'll agree that it's a delicious synergy far greater than the sum of its parts. Serve this dish plain or spoon over cooked brown rice or whole-grain couscous.

PREP TIME: 10 minutes
COOK TIME: 23 minutes

INGREDIENTS | SERVES 6

1½ teaspoons olive oil

1 large onion, peeled and diced

4 cloves garlic, minced

2 (15-ounce) cans no salt added diced tomatoes, with juice

2 medium potatoes, peeled and diced

2 cups vegetable broth

2 medium carrots, peeled and sliced

½ pound white-fleshed fish, cut into 1" chunks

1 jalapeño pepper, seeded and minced

1 bay leaf

¼ pound small shrimp, peeled

⅓ cup chopped fresh cilantro

½ teaspoon grated orange zest

½ teaspoon freshly ground black pepper

1. Heat oil in a small stockpot over medium heat. Add onion and garlic and cook, stirring, 3 minutes, until they begin to sweat.

2. Add tomatoes with juice, potatoes, broth, carrots, fish, jalapeño, and bay leaf and stir to combine. Cover the pot and cook, stirring occasionally, 15 minutes.

3. Add shrimp, cilantro, orange zest, and pepper and stir well. Simmer until shrimp are pink, 3–5 minutes, then remove from heat.

4. Remove bay leaf and serve immediately.

PER SERVING Calories: 191 | Fat: 5.4 g | Protein: 12.8 g | Sodium: 513 mg | Fiber: 4.1 g | Carbohydrates: 23.2 g | Sugar: 7.6 g

Slow Cooker Split Pea Soup

Unlike dried beans, split peas require no presoaking, so you can assemble this dish any morning and enjoy dinner later in the day. Split peas are high in iron and magnesium, low in fat and sodium, and high in fiber and protein, making this an energy-boosting, metabolism-maintaining, healthy blood-building bowl of MIND diet goodness.

PREP TIME: 10 minutes
COOK TIME: 7 hours

INGREDIENTS | SERVES 8

1 medium onion, peeled and diced

2 medium carrots, peeled and diced

2 medium stalks celery, trimmed and diced

2 medium potatoes, peeled and diced

1 pound (2¼ cups) dry green split peas, rinsed

7 cups vegetable broth

1 bay leaf

2 teaspoons all-purpose seasoning

1 teaspoon ground coriander

½ teaspoon ground cumin

½ teaspoon freshly ground black pepper

1. Place all ingredients in a slow cooker and stir to combine. Cover, set to high, and cook, stirring occasionally, 7 hours.

2. Remove bay leaf and serve hot.

PER SERVING Calories: 252 | Fat: 0.6 g | Protein: 14.5 g | Sodium: 851 mg | Fiber: 15.6 g | Carbohydrates: 48.8 g | Sugar: 7.8 g

All-Purpose Seasoning

If there's a single seasoning you'll want to find for your diet, it's this one! All-purpose seasoning is a unique blend of herbs, spices, dehydrated vegetables, citrus zest, and sometimes nutritional yeast. Its combination of flavors can replace salt both at the table and in recipes. Benson's Table Tasty is a completely natural, salt-free blend with a salty flavor. It contains no potassium chloride or other chemicals and is sold online.

Slow Cooker Lentil and Quinoa Chili

Lentils and quinoa are so comforting, healthy, and inexpensive, they merit addition to all sorts of things, including this magnificently different take on chili. If you don't have ground cinnamon, use a cinnamon stick instead; just remember to remove before eating! Vegetable juice may be substituted for the broth for another fabulous dimension of flavor. Serve hot spooned over baked potatoes for a complete low-fat, vegan, and gluten-free meal.

PREP TIME: 10 minutes
COOK TIME: 6 hours

INGREDIENTS | SERVES 8

1 medium onion, peeled and diced

3 cloves garlic, minced

1 medium red bell pepper, seeded and diced

2 (15-ounce) cans no salt added diced tomatoes, with juice

1 (15-ounce) can black beans, drained and rinsed

1 (15-ounce) can kidney beans, drained and rinsed

1 cup dried lentils, rinsed

½ cup uncooked quinoa, rinsed

3 cups vegetable broth

1 tablespoon chili seasoning

1 teaspoon ground cumin

¼ teaspoon curry powder

⅛ teaspoon ground cinnamon

½ teaspoon freshly ground black pepper

½ cup chopped fresh cilantro

1 ripe avocado, pitted and diced

1. Place all ingredients except cilantro and avocado in a slow cooker and stir well to combine. Cover, set to high, and cook 6 hours, stirring occasionally if possible.

2. At the end of cooking time, remove lid and stir in cilantro. Spoon chili into bowls and top with avocado.

3. Serve immediately.

PER SERVING Calories: 280 | Fat: 3.5 g | Protein: 15.6 g | Sodium: 578 mg | Fiber: 13.2 g | Carbohydrates: 48.1 g | Sugar: 6.6 g

An Important Note about Quinoa

Quinoa has a bitter-tasting outer coating on its grains that must be removed prior to cooking. Most brands of commercial quinoa remove this prior to packaging, so you can simply measure and cook. But if you're not using organic prewashed quinoa, don't forget to rinse well prior to cooking.

Chili Con Carne for a Crowd

Whether it's a family get-together, poker night with friends, or a Super Bowl block party, this slow-cooked chili has you covered. Ground turkey lends heft and flavor to the vegetable base, but with lower cholesterol and fat than ground beef, making this a much healthier alternative. Serve the chili over baked potatoes or brown rice, or use it as a delicious topping for nachos. For a smaller group, simply halve the recipe.

PREP TIME: 15 minutes
COOK TIME: 4–8 hours

INGREDIENTS | SERVES 10

1 pound lean (fat-free) ground turkey

2 large onions, peeled and chopped

4 cloves garlic, minced

2 medium bell peppers, seeded and diced

2 (15-ounce) cans no salt added diced tomatoes, with juice

1 (8-ounce) can tomato sauce

1 (15-ounce) can kidney beans, drained and rinsed

1 (15-ounce) can pinto beans, drained and rinsed

1 tablespoon agave nectar

1 tablespoon apple cider vinegar

1 tablespoon low-sodium soy sauce

1 tablespoon chili seasoning

2 teaspoons ground cumin

1 teaspoon dried oregano

½ teaspoon ground coriander

¼ teaspoon dried red pepper flakes

½ teaspoon freshly ground black pepper

¼ cup chopped fresh cilantro

1. Heat a nonstick skillet over medium heat. Add ground turkey, onions, and garlic and cook, stirring, until turkey is no longer pink, about 5 minutes. Remove from heat and transfer contents to a slow cooker.

2. Add remaining ingredients except cilantro to the slow cooker and stir well. Cover and cook on high 4–5 hours or on low 6–8 hours, stirring occasionally if possible.

3. Just before serving stir in cilantro. Serve hot.

PER SERVING Calories: 170 | Fat: 1.3 g | Protein: 16.9 g | Sodium: 371 mg | Fiber: 6.5 g | Carbohydrates: 23.7 g | Sugar: 7.1 g

Chicken Soup with Jalapeño and Lime

Set your taste buds abuzz with the zing of fresh lime! This soup is brimming with flavor, yet nearly fat-free. For added heft, ladle soup over bowls of cooked brown or wild rice, wide noodles, or quinoa. To reduce the amount of heat, remove the seeds from the jalapeño. If you are particularly sensitive, wear disposable gloves while mincing the pepper, and be sure not to touch your face, nose, or eyes.

PREP TIME: 10 minutes
COOK TIME: 15 minutes

INGREDIENTS | SERVES 8

2 cups shredded, cooked chicken

1 medium red onion, peeled and diced

3 cloves garlic, minced

2 medium carrots, peeled and sliced

1 medium stalk celery, trimmed and sliced

1 medium red bell pepper, seeded and diced

1 jalapeño pepper, seeded and minced

1 (15-ounce) can no salt added diced tomatoes, with juice

Juice of 2 medium limes

8 cups chicken broth

1 teaspoon ground cumin

½ teaspoon ground coriander

¼ teaspoon dried oregano

½ teaspoon freshly ground black pepper

2 tablespoons chopped fresh cilantro

1 medium lime, cut into 8 wedges

1. Place all ingredients except cilantro and lime in a large stockpot and bring to a boil over high heat.

2. Reduce heat to low, cover, and simmer 15 minutes.

3. Remove from heat, ladle into bowls, and garnish with cilantro and lime wedges. Serve immediately.

PER SERVING Calories: 99 | Fat: 1.4 g | Protein: 12.1 g | Sodium: 978 mg | Fiber: 2.0 g | Carbohydrates: 8.4 g | Sugar: 4.7 g

Squeeze Your Citrus

To get the most out of citrus fruit, give it a squeeze! Before juicing, roll citrus on the counter, pressing down firmly with your hands. The pressure will allow more of the juice to be extracted, and it'll make your hands smell great, too! Another tip: when citrus gets old, it often dries out inside. Microwave older fruit for 15 seconds to get the most juice from your squeeze.

Slow Cooker Irish Bean and Cabbage Stew

This stew is simple, inexpensive, and supremely healthy, and most importantly it's delicious. Because your slow cooker does all the work (save for chopping), it's a terrific dish for a busy day. The recipe calls for pinto beans, but you can use whichever bean you like best. The bright flavor of fresh parsley is the perfect finishing touch, so don't skimp!

PREP TIME: 15 minutes
COOK TIME: 6–8 hours

INGREDIENTS | SERVES 8

1 medium onion, peeled and diced

2 medium stalks celery, trimmed and diced

3 cloves garlic, minced

½ medium head cabbage, chopped

1 pound red potatoes, diced

1 (15-ounce) can pinto beans, drained and rinsed

1 (15-ounce) can no salt added diced tomatoes, with juice

⅓ cup dry pearl barley

1 bay leaf

1 teaspoon dried thyme

½ teaspoon caraway seeds

½ teaspoon dried rosemary, crushed

½ teaspoon freshly ground black pepper

6 cups vegetable broth

¼ cup chopped fresh parsley

1. Place all ingredients except parsley in a slow cooker and stir to combine. Cover, set to low, and cook 6–8 hours, stirring occasionally if possible.

2. Ladle into bowls and sprinkle with fresh parsley. Serve hot.

PER SERVING Calories: 152 | Fat: 0.4 g | Protein: 6.0 g | Sodium: 835 mg | Fiber: 6.8 g | Carbohydrates: 33.0 g | Sugar: 6.4 g

CHAPTER 10

Vegetables and Sides

Sweet and Spicy Brussels Sprouts

These Sweet and Spicy Brussels Sprouts are the best Brussels sprouts ever. Spicy, sweet, tangy, and absolutely irresistible, the combination of flavors in the caramelized sprouts will keep you reaching for more . . . and more. Feel free to double the recipe; even then, you may not get enough.

PREP TIME: 5 minutes
COOK TIME: 35 minutes

INGREDIENTS | SERVES 8

2 pounds fresh Brussels sprouts, trimmed and larger ones halved

1 tablespoon agave nectar

1 tablespoon lime juice

1 tablespoon low-sodium soy sauce

1 tablespoon olive oil

1 tablespoon sriracha

½ teaspoon freshly ground black pepper

Tell Me More about Sriracha

Sriracha is a spicy red chili sauce made from chili peppers, distilled vinegar, garlic, sugar, and salt. Originally from Thailand, it's become one of the most popular condiments in the world. Even a tiny bit will add a lot of flavor, not to mention heat, to many dishes. Look for it in the Asian section of most supermarkets. It's sold under several name brands; a top seller is Huy Fong, which has a rooster on the bottle.

1. Preheat oven to 400°F. Line a baking sheet with parchment and set aside.

2. Place Brussels sprouts in a medium mixing bowl.

3. Measure agave, lime juice, oil, soy sauce, and sriracha into a small mixing bowl and whisk well to combine. Pour mixture over Brussels sprouts and toss well to coat.

4. Spread Brussels sprouts in a single layer on the parchment and sprinkle with pepper. Place sheet on middle rack in oven and bake 35 minutes until tender.

5. Remove sheet from oven. Serve immediately.

PER SERVING Calories: 62 | Fat: 1.9 g | Protein: 3.1 g | Sodium: 115 mg | Fiber: 3.4 g | Carbohydrates: 10.3 g | Sugar: 4.2 g

Perfect Steamed Broccoli

People who dislike broccoli might not hate the vegetable itself; they might just resent the way it's prepared. Here's a foolproof recipe for making perfectly crisp, perfectly seasoned broccoli every time. The trick? The broccoli is steamed gently in a small amount of vegetable broth instead of plain water. The flavor of the broth permeates the spears, leaving them tasty and tender.

PREP TIME: 5 minutes
COOK TIME: 10 minutes

INGREDIENTS | SERVES 4

½ cup vegetable broth
1½ pounds broccoli spears
½ teaspoon freshly ground black pepper

1. Place a large sauté pan over medium-high heat. Add broth, then arrange broccoli evenly in the pan. Cover the pan and set a kitchen timer to 7 minutes.

2. Stir broccoli once or twice while cooking, then check spears after 7 minutes for doneness. If tender, remove from heat immediately. If still a bit too crisp, cover pan and check every minute; cook no more than 10 minutes total.

3. Remove from heat and sprinkle with pepper. Serve immediately.

PER SERVING Calories: 58 | Fat: 0.1 g | Protein: 4.8 g | Sodium: 103 mg | Fiber: 4.5 g | Carbohydrates: 11.6 g | Sugar: 3.0 g

Five-Spice Fried Rice

The key to making perfect fried rice is to use cold rice only—so this is a great way to use up leftover rice. Make the recipe as written, or use whatever protein and vegetables you have on hand, even cubed fruit, like pineapple or mango. Serve with chopped cashews or peanuts and sliced green onion.

PREP TIME: 5 minutes
COOK TIME: 10 minutes

INGREDIENTS | SERVES 6

2 teaspoons olive oil

1 medium onion, peeled and diced

3 cloves garlic, minced

2 medium carrots, peeled and diced

4 cups cold cooked brown rice

1 cup frozen green peas

1½ tablespoons low-sodium soy sauce

1 tablespoon natural (unflavored) rice wine vinegar

1 teaspoon sriracha

½ teaspoon ground ginger

¼ teaspoon five-spice powder

½ teaspoon freshly ground black pepper

1. Heat oil in a wok or large sauté pan over medium heat. Add onion, garlic, and carrots and cook, stirring, 5 minutes.

2. Add remaining ingredients and stir well to coat. Cook, stirring, 5 minutes until rice is fragrant and vegetables are tender.

3. Remove from heat and serve immediately.

PER SERVING Calories: 198 | Fat: 2.6 g | Protein: 5.5 g | Sodium: 181 mg | Fiber: 4.8 g | Carbohydrates: 38.1 g | Sugar: 3.6 g

What Is Five-Spice Powder?

Five-spice powder is a flavorfully fragrant blend of cinnamon, cloves, star anise, pepper, and fennel. It's sold in many supermarkets and specialty food stores; if you can't find it, make your own. Combine 1 teaspoon ground cinnamon, 1 teaspoon anise seed or 1 star anise, ¼ teaspoon fennel seed, ¼ teaspoon ground black pepper, and ⅛ teaspoon ground cloves. Pulse into a powder using a small spice grinder or mortar and pestle. This yields a tablespoon; you only need a ¼ teaspoon for this recipe. Sealed in a clean lidded jar or plastic bag, the excess spice mixture should remain fresh for 2 years.

Roasted Lemon Asparagus

In this recipe, fresh asparagus is tossed with lemon juice and a tiny bit of oil, then oven roasted. What sounds so simple becomes an extraordinarily delicious side dish, full of citrus flavor and complexity.

PREP TIME: 5 minutes
COOK TIME: 20 minutes

INGREDIENTS | SERVES 6

1½ pounds fresh asparagus, washed, trimmed, and cut into 3" pieces
2 tablespoons lemon juice
1 teaspoon olive oil
½ teaspoon freshly ground black pepper

Roasting for Flavor

Roasting is simply cooking food at a very high temperature. You can roast in an oven, or you can roast over an open flame. Oven roasting allows for convenience and control. You're able to adjust not only the temperature of the oven but the proximity of the food to the flame. The roasting process allows the natural sugars present in many foods to caramelize, leaving the cooked versions much sweeter and more complex than they were when raw.

1. Preheat oven to 425°F. Line a baking sheet with parchment and set aside.

2. Put asparagus in a medium mixing bowl and add lemon juice, oil, and pepper. Toss gently to coat.

3. Spread asparagus in a single layer on the baking sheet. Place the baking sheet on the middle rack in the oven and roast until tender, 20 minutes.

4. Remove pan from oven. Serve immediately.

PER SERVING Calories: 30 | Fat: 0.8 g | Protein: 2.5 g | Sodium: 2 mg | Fiber: 2.5 g | Carbohydrates: 4.9 g | Sugar: 2.3 g

Butternut Squash with Brown Sugar and Walnuts

Butternut squash is a gorgeous way to brighten any meal. Here, its natural sweetness is heightened with brown sugar and cinnamon. The flavor pairs wonderfully with poultry, making this an ideal side for the holidays. Serve with your choice of dark leafy greens and cooked whole grains for a healthy, balanced meal. For a different twist on the same dish, use sweet potatoes and pecans and reduce the cooking time by 10 minutes.

PREP TIME: 10 minutes
COOK TIME: 45 minutes

INGREDIENTS | SERVES 6

6 cups cubed butternut squash
1 tablespoon olive oil
¼ cup brown sugar (unpacked)
¼ cup walnuts
1 teaspoon ground cinnamon

1. Preheat oven to 425°F. Line a baking sheet with parchment and set aside.

2. Place squash in a large mixing bowl. Add remaining ingredients and toss well to coat.

3. Arrange squash on the baking pan. Place pan on the middle rack in oven and bake until tender, 45 minutes.

4. Remove from oven and serve immediately.

PER SERVING Calories: 133 | Fat: 4.9 g | Protein: 2.1 g | Sodium: 7 mg | Fiber: 3.3 g | Carbohydrates: 23.2 g | Sugar: 9.1 g

Oven-Baked Sweet Potato Fries

These versatile potato wedges can be served with a myriad of main courses and adapted to suit any taste. Vary the flavor of the seasoning for interest: Southwestern, lemon-pepper, all-purpose, Jamaican jerk, and so on. For a sweeter version, toss with 2 tablespoons brown sugar and ½ teaspoon ground cinnamon. Serve with ketchup or homemade vegan mayonnaise mixed with a little sriracha.

PREP TIME: 10 minutes
COOK TIME: 35 minutes

INGREDIENTS | SERVES 4

4 medium sweet potatoes, peeled and cut into wedges
1 tablespoon olive oil
1 teaspoon all-purpose seasoning
½ teaspoon freshly ground black pepper

Sweet Potato Facts

Sweet potatoes are a staple anyone on the MIND diet should embrace. They're inexpensive and extremely versatile, adapting to almost any type of cuisine. They're high in vitamins A, B_6, and C; contain beta carotene, magnesium, calcium, iron, protein, and fiber; and are super low in sodium. When buying sweet potatoes, look for firm orange flesh, free of soft spots or blemishes. At home, store them in a dark cabinet or drawer, never in the refrigerator.

1. Preheat oven to 425°F. Line a baking sheet with parchment and set aside.

2. Place sweet potatoes in a large mixing bowl and add oil, seasoning, and pepper; toss well to coat.

3. Arrange wedges on the baking sheet. Place the baking sheet on the middle rack in oven and bake 20 minutes. Flip wedges, then return to oven and bake another 15 minutes until tender.

4. Remove from oven and serve immediately.

PER SERVING Calories: 119 | Fat: 3.3 g | Protein: 1.7 g | Sodium: 57 mg | Fiber: 3.2 g | Carbohydrates: 21.1 g | Sugar: 4.4 g

Baked Spinach and Pea Risotto

There's something magical about the combination of tastes and textures in this risotto. The wine, broth, and cheese lend so much flavor, and the creaminess keeps you coming back for more. Vegans can eliminate the cheese altogether—the risotto will be just as delicious without it. If you're looking to replace the wine, substitute ¼ cup vegetable broth plus 2–3 tablespoons white wine vinegar.

PREP TIME: 5 minutes
COOK TIME: 25 minutes

INGREDIENTS | SERVES 6

1 tablespoon olive oil
1 medium shallot, peeled and chopped
½ teaspoon freshly ground black pepper
½ cup dry white wine
3 cups vegetable broth
1 cup uncooked Arborio rice
1 cup frozen peas, thawed
2 cups chopped fresh baby spinach
¼ cup grated Parmesan cheese

Hidden Substances in Frozen Vegetables

Many frozen vegetables are just that, frozen vegetables. But others contain things you don't want, like added salt and sauces. When selecting frozen vegetables, check nutrition facts carefully to ensure you're buying the vegetables you want, without anything else.

1. Preheat oven to 425°F.

2. Place a Dutch oven or similar lidded casserole pan on the stovetop over medium-high heat. Add oil, shallot, and pepper and sauté 3 minutes.

3. Add wine and cook, stirring, until almost evaporated, 2 minutes.

4. Stir in broth and rice and bring to a boil, then cover the pot and transfer to the middle rack in the oven. Bake 20 minutes until rice is tender and creamy.

5. Remove from oven. Add peas, spinach, and cheese and stir well to combine. Serve immediately.

PER SERVING Calories: 204 | Fat: 3.4 g | Protein: 5.1 g | Sodium: 573 mg | Fiber: 1.8 g | Carbohydrates: 33.8 g | Sugar: 2.7 g

Garlicky Green Beans

This dish is simple enough for you to prepare daily, and you'll never tire of eating these beans, either straight from the pan or on a plate for dinner. For larger parties or holidays, double the recipe, but make the beans a pound at a time; they won't cook perfectly if overcrowded in the pan.

PREP TIME: 5 minutes
COOK TIME: 10 minutes

INGREDIENTS | SERVES 4

1 cup water

1 pound fresh green beans, washed and trimmed

2 teaspoons olive oil

4 cloves garlic, minced

½ teaspoon all-purpose seasoning

½ teaspoon freshly ground black pepper

1. Heat water in a large sauté pan over medium heat. Add green beans and stir to coat. Cook, stirring frequently, 5 minutes.

2. Remove pan from heat and drain beans into a large colander. Rinse beans under cold water.

3. Return pan to medium heat, add oil and garlic, and cook, stirring, 1–2 minutes. Add beans and cook, stirring, just until tender, 2–3 minutes.

4. Remove from heat and sprinkle with seasoning and pepper. Serve immediately.

PER SERVING Calories: 59 | Fat: 2.3 g | Protein: 2.3 g | Sodium: 9 mg | Fiber: 4.0 g | Carbohydrates: 9.1 g | Sugar: 0.0 g

Southwestern Corn Sauté

The perfect partner for taco night, this speedy side might be the star of the show. A can of black or pinto beans easily transforms this into a burrito filling; a can of diced tomatoes makes it an extra-hearty warm salsa for spooning over nachos or serving with tortilla chips. No need to thaw the frozen corn; it cooks fully in the pan.

PREP TIME: 10 minutes
COOK TIME: 10 minutes

INGREDIENTS | SERVES 6

2 teaspoons olive oil

1 medium red onion, peeled and diced

1 medium green bell pepper, seeded and diced

1 medium red bell pepper, seeded and diced

3 cups frozen corn

3 cloves garlic, minced

2 tablespoons lime juice

1 teaspoon agave nectar

1 teaspoon ground cumin

½ teaspoon dried oregano

½ teaspoon chili seasoning

⅛ teaspoon ground cayenne

1 ripe avocado, pitted and diced

¼ cup chopped fresh cilantro

½ teaspoon freshly ground black pepper

1. Heat oil in a large sauté pan over medium heat. Add onion and cook, stirring, 2 minutes.

2. Add peppers and cook, stirring, 3 minutes.

3. Add corn, garlic, lime juice, agave, cumin, oregano, chili seasoning, and cayenne and stir well to combine. Cook, stirring frequently, 5 minutes.

4. Remove from heat. Stir in avocado, cilantro, and black pepper.

5. Serve immediately.

PER SERVING Calories: 139 | Fat: 5.2 g | Protein: 3.2 g | Sodium: 13 mg | Fiber: 4.6 g | Carbohydrates: 23.1 g | Sugar: 5.1 g

Avocado Facts

Avocados are native to South and Central America and are actually a fruit, not a vegetable. Ripe avocados have a smooth, leathery skin that when ripe yields to pressure. The easiest way to prepare a ripe avocado is to cut lengthwise through the fruit to the core, gently break open, remove the pit, and peel away the skin. Avocados are high in vitamins B_6, C, E, and K, and have been shown to protect against prostate cancer.

Coconut Quinoa with Kale

Warm, comforting, and filled with yummy flavor, this quinoa "pilaf" is reminiscent of couscous. But even if you dislike both coconut and quinoa, you're guaranteed to love this speedy side! Try it for yourself; it may become a favorite, too.

PREP TIME: 5 minutes
COOK TIME: 25 minutes

INGREDIENTS | SERVES 4

1 cup uncooked quinoa

1 (15-ounce) can light coconut milk, divided

¼ cup chopped fresh cilantro

1 teaspoon olive oil

1 medium onion, peeled and diced

3 cloves garlic, minced

4 cups chopped fresh kale leaves

1½ teaspoons agave nectar

1½ teaspoons apple cider vinegar

1½ teaspoons lime juice

1½ teaspoons low-sodium soy sauce

½ teaspoon freshly ground black pepper

1. Place quinoa in a fine-mesh sieve and rinse under cold water for a minute or two. Transfer quinoa to a medium saucepan, add 1 cup coconut milk, and stir to combine.

2. Bring to a boil over medium-high heat; then lower the heat to medium-low, cover, and simmer 15 minutes. Remove from heat, uncover, and fluff quinoa. Add cilantro and toss to combine. Set aside.

3. Heat oil in a large sauté pan over medium heat. Add onion and garlic and cook, stirring, 2 minutes. Add kale, agave, vinegar, lime juice, and soy sauce and stir to combine. Cook, stirring frequently, 8 minutes or until most of the liquid has evaporated.

4. Remove from heat, add quinoa, and stir to combine. Add pepper and serve immediately.

PER SERVING Calories: 263 | Fat: 9.6 g | Protein: 7.3 g | Sodium: 76 mg | Fiber: 4.2 g | Carbohydrates: 35.5 g | Sugar: 3.4 g

Pan-Roasted Radishes with Figs and Greens

These Pan-Roasted Radishes with Figs and Greens are so simple and so good! Cooked radishes have a milder flavor than their raw counterparts. Here they're browned until tender, then tossed with plumped figs, pecans, and fresh greens. If you enjoy radish greens, substitute an equal amount for the arugula.

PREP TIME: 10 minutes
COOK TIME: 12 minutes

INGREDIENTS | SERVES 6

1 cup water
½ cup sliced dried Mission figs
2 tablespoons olive oil, divided
2 cups (10 ounces) trimmed radishes, halved or quartered
8 cups fresh baby spinach
4 cups fresh arugula
¼ cup chopped pecans
¼ cup chopped olives
2 teaspoons balsamic vinegar
½ teaspoon freshly ground black pepper

Radish Facts

Radishes originated in China and were first brought to North America by early colonists in the 1600s. They're a member of the *Brassica* (cabbage) genus and are related to kale, broccoli, and cauliflower. Radishes are a quick and easy-growing crop, perfect for any home garden. All of the plant is edible, both the leaves and root, and can be eaten raw or cooked. Radishes come in many shapes and sizes and vary in flavor from almost sweet to distinctly sharp and spicy. Their pungent flavor mellows with cooking. Radishes are low in calories, high in vitamin C, antioxidants, minerals, and fiber.

1. Place water in a kettle, microwave-safe bowl, or small saucepan and heat until boiling.

2. Place figs in a small bowl and cover with boiling water. Set aside 5 minutes to plump, then drain.

3. Heat 1 tablespoon oil in a large sauté pan over medium-high heat. Add radishes, cover, and cook undisturbed 3 minutes until brown on one side. Uncover, shake pan, and cook another 3–4 minutes until radishes are tender. Remove from heat, place radishes in a bowl, and set aside.

4. Return pan to heat and add the remaining 1 tablespoon oil. Add spinach and arugula and cook while stirring with tongs until barely wilted, about 2 minutes.

5. Add figs, pecans, olives, and radishes. Cover the pan and cook 3 minutes until everything is heated through.

6. Remove from heat, uncover, and drizzle with balsamic vinegar. Add pepper and serve immediately.

PER SERVING Calories: 128 | Fat: 8.4 g | Protein: 2.6 g | Sodium: 93 mg | Fiber: 3.6 g | Carbohydrates: 12.7 g | Sugar: 8.4 g

Red Potatoes with Mustard, Peas, and Parsley

In this recipe, simple peas and potatoes are elevated to new heights with the addition of mustard, wine, and onion. Add a couple of chopped hard-boiled eggs or a cup of cooked beans for extra protein if desired.

PREP TIME: 10 minutes
COOK TIME: 17 minutes

INGREDIENTS | SERVES 4

1½ pounds red potatoes, scrubbed and cut into 1½" cubes

1 cup frozen peas

¼ cup dry white wine

1 small onion, peeled and chopped

2 tablespoons mustard

1 tablespoon olive oil

½ teaspoon freshly ground black pepper

¼ cup chopped fresh parsley

1. Place potatoes in a large pot, add enough water to cover by an inch, and bring to a boil over high heat. Boil until tender, roughly 15 minutes. Add frozen peas to the pot during the last 2–3 minutes of cooking.

2. Drain potatoes and peas into a colander and set aside. Do not wash the pot.

3. Return the pot to the stove, place over high heat, and add wine and onion. Cook 2 minutes to soften, then remove pot from the heat and whisk in mustard, oil, and pepper.

4. Add potatoes and peas back into the pot and toss well to coat. Add parsley and stir to combine. Serve immediately.

PER SERVING Calories: 184 | Fat: 3.8 g | Protein: 5.3 g | Sodium: 242 mg | Fiber: 5.4 g | Carbohydrates: 30.9 g | Sugar: 4.9 g

Oven-Roasted Cherry Tomatoes

Roasting is the magic hat of cooking. Just pop a food into the oven and out comes pure deliciousness. In this recipe cherry tomatoes are rendered irresistible with little more than a lot of heat. This recipe works wonderfully not only with ripe red tomatoes but with unripe green tomatoes too. It's a great way to use and enjoy everything nature provides.

PREP TIME: 5 minutes
COOK TIME: 45–60 minutes

INGREDIENTS | SERVES 4

4 cups fresh cherry tomatoes, washed
1 tablespoon olive oil
1 teaspoon all-purpose seasoning
½ teaspoon garlic powder
¼ teaspoon dried thyme
¼ teaspoon freshly ground black pepper

The Many Uses of Oven-Roasted Tomatoes

In addition to being eaten plain, roasted tomatoes can be used as a topping for tacos or burritos; as a filling for wrap sandwiches; as a stand-in for canned tomatoes in your favorite soup, stew, or chili; as a base for pasta sauce; as a base for salsa verde; and more!

1. Preheat oven to 425°F. Line a sided baking sheet with parchment and set aside.

2. Place tomatoes in a medium mixing bowl. Add remaining ingredients and toss well to coat.

3. Place tomatoes on the baking sheet; roll gently to arrange in a single layer. Place baking sheet on middle rack in oven and bake 45–60 minutes until tomatoes are nicely deflated and juicy.

4. Remove from oven. Serve hot or cold. Store leftovers in the refrigerator up to 3 days and add to recipes or consume as desired.

PER SERVING Calories: 58 | Fat: 3.5 g | Protein: 1.4 g | Sodium: 7 mg | Fiber: 1.9 g | Carbohydrates: 6.2 g | Sugar: 3.9 g

Carrots with Indian Spices

Lively and flavorful, this side dish is a great partner for curries or grilled meat. For more spice, add half of a minced jalapeño pepper along with the other seasonings.

PREP TIME: 10 minutes
COOK TIME: 11 minutes

INGREDIENTS | SERVES 6

1 tablespoon minced fresh ginger

1½ teaspoons mustard seeds

1 teaspoon freshly ground black pepper

½ teaspoon ground coriander

½ teaspoon ground cumin

¼ teaspoon curry powder

¼ cup water

1 tablespoon olive oil

2 pounds fresh carrots, peeled and cut diagonally into ½" slices

Juice of 1 medium lime

¼ cup chopped fresh cilantro

1. Measure ginger, mustard seeds, pepper, coriander, cumin, and curry powder into a small bowl. Mix and set aside.

2. Place a sauté pan over medium heat. Add water, oil, and carrots to the pan and bring to a boil. Cover pan and cook, shaking occasionally, until carrots are just barely tender, about 7 minutes.

3. Uncover the pan and continue to cook until carrots begin to sizzle in the oil, about 2 minutes.

4. Add spice mixture and cook stirring continuously 2 minutes.

5. Remove pan from heat. Add lime juice and cilantro and stir to combine. Serve immediately.

PER SERVING Calories: 87 | Fat: 2.7 g | Protein: 1.7 g | Sodium: 104 mg | Fiber: 4.6 g | Carbohydrates: 15.7 g | Sugar: 7.3 g

Oven-Baked Mushroom Barley Pilaf

This creamy pilaf filled with the earthy flavors of mushrooms and barley is warm comfort food at its best. Easy serving and wide appeal make this a great potluck dish, especially in the winter, and the hands-off oven baking makes cooking a breeze.

PREP TIME: 10 minutes
COOK TIME: 1 hour 10 minutes

INGREDIENTS | SERVES 6

2 tablespoons olive oil

10 ounces fresh mushrooms, chopped

1 medium onion, peeled and chopped

4 cloves garlic, minced

¼ cup chopped walnuts

½ cup red wine

1 cup uncooked pearl barley

3 cups vegetable broth

1 bay leaf

1 teaspoon all-purpose seasoning

½ teaspoon dried basil

¼ teaspoon dried thyme

¼ teaspoon dried marjoram

¼ teaspoon freshly ground black pepper

¼ cup chopped fresh parsley

1. Preheat oven to 350°F.

2. Heat oil in a Dutch oven or similar lidded casserole. Add mushrooms, onion, and garlic and cook, stirring, 5 minutes.

3. Add walnuts, wine, barley, broth, bay leaf, seasoning, basil, thyme, marjoram, and pepper and cook, stirring frequently, 5 minutes.

4. Cover the pot and transfer to the middle rack in the oven. Bake 1 hour until barley is tender.

5. Remove from oven. Carefully remove bay leaf and discard. Stir in parsley and serve immediately.

PER SERVING Calories: 231 | Fat: 7.9 g | Protein: 5.9 g | Sodium: 478 mg | Fiber: 6.5 g | Carbohydrates: 32.6 g | Sugar: 3.2 g

Mushroom Facts

Mushrooms are extremely low in fat and calories, and are a great source of copper, selenium, B vitamins, and antioxidants. Mushrooms have been shown to boost immunity against infection, inhibit cancer, reduce inflammation, and protect against cardiovascular and other diseases. At home, store fresh mushrooms in the refrigerator; the cold inhibits discoloration and helps maintain their phytonutrient content.

Roasted Beets with Chili-Lime Vinaigrette

*This delicious side will appeal to even the staunchest of beet haters.
The natural sweetness of the beets is accentuated by oven roasting;
the tender beets are then tossed with ripe orange, mango, and
almonds and drizzled with a stellar spicy-citrus vinaigrette.*

PREP TIME: 15 minutes
COOK TIME: 60 minutes

INGREDIENTS | SERVES 4

2 medium beets, trimmed and washed

4 cups mixed salad greens

1 large orange, peeled and cut into bite-sized chunks

1 ripe mango, peeled, cored, and diced

¼ cup slivered almonds

3 tablespoons lime juice

1 tablespoon apple cider vinegar

2 teaspoons agave nectar

3 tablespoons olive oil

1 teaspoon mustard

1 teaspoon ground cumin

½ teaspoon chili seasoning

1. Preheat oven to 400°F.

2. Wrap beets tightly in aluminum foil. Place in oven and roast 1 hour, until tender. Remove from oven and cool to the touch. The skins should slip off; if not, gently peel them. Cut beets into bite-sized pieces. Note: beets may be roasted a day ahead and kept wrapped in the refrigerator.

3. Place greens in a large serving bowl, then add beets, orange, mango, and almonds and toss well to combine. Set aside.

4. In a small bowl, combine lime juice, vinegar, agave, oil, mustard, cumin, and chili seasoning; whisk well to combine.

5. Pour vinaigrette over fruit and vegetables and toss well to coat. Serve immediately.

PER SERVING Calories: 230 | Fat: 13.5 g | Protein: 3.8 g | Sodium: 84 mg | Fiber: 5.0 g | Carbohydrates: 28.0 g | Sugar: 20.9 g

Swiss Chard with Apples, Raisins, and Pecans

In this recipe the sweetness of the apples and raisins tempers the bitterness of the greens, rendering them addictively delicious. For variety, substitute kale or beet greens for the chard, and walnuts and dried cranberries for the pecans and raisins.

PREP TIME: 15 minutes
COOK TIME: 10 minutes

INGREDIENTS | SERVES 8

½ cup water

¼ cup seedless raisins

2 tablespoons olive oil

1 medium red onion, peeled and diced

1½ pounds fresh Swiss chard, stems removed and sliced, leaves chopped

2 large Honeycrisp apples, peeled, cored, and diced

½ cup chopped pecans

1 tablespoon low-sodium soy sauce

1 tablespoon apple cider vinegar

2 teaspoons agave nectar

½ teaspoon freshly ground black pepper

Swiss Chard Facts

Swiss chard is a dark leafy green with colorful stalks akin to celery. It has a somewhat bitter taste that mellows with cooking, and is particularly well suited to sautéing with a little olive oil and garlic. Swiss chard is an excellent source of vitamins A, C, and K, plus manganese, potassium, iron, fiber, and antioxidants, and has been linked to the prevention of Alzheimer's, cancer, and cardiovascular disease.

1. Place water in a kettle, microwave-safe bowl, or small saucepan and heat until boiling.

2. Place raisins in a small bowl and add boiling water to cover. Set aside to plump.

3. Heat oil in a large sauté pan over medium heat. Add onion and cook, stirring, 2 minutes. Add chard stems and apple and cook, stirring, 2 minutes, until they begin to sweat.

4. Drain raisins and reserve 1 tablespoon soaking water. Add raisins and water to the pan along with chard leaves and stir well to combine. Cover the pan and cook 6 minutes until chard is wilted and tender.

5. Uncover the pan and stir briefly to release any extra liquid. Add remaining ingredients and stir well to combine.

6. Remove from heat and serve immediately.

PER SERVING Calories: 96 | Fat: 3.5 g | Protein: 2.1 g | Sodium: 246 mg | Fiber: 2.6 g | Carbohydrates: 16.3 g | Sugar: 10.9 g

CHAPTER 11

Beans and Legumes

Coconut Collards with Sweet Potatoes and Black Beans

Talk about fantastic flavor! In this recipe the collards are bathed with a subtle sweetness from the coconut milk, sweet potatoes, carrots, and tomatoes, and a light citrus kick from the lime juice and curry paste lends the perfect finish. For a spicier version, add a fresh minced jalapeño pepper or ¼ teaspoon ground cayenne while cooking.

PREP TIME: 15 minutes
COOK TIME: 23 minutes

INGREDIENTS | SERVES 8

1 tablespoon olive oil

1 medium onion, peeled and chopped

4 cloves garlic, minced

2 medium carrots, peeled and sliced

2 medium stalks celery, trimmed and sliced

1 medium red bell pepper, seeded and diced

2 medium sweet potatoes, peeled and cubed

1 pound collard greens, chopped

1 (15-ounce) can no salt added diced tomatoes, with juice

1 (15-ounce) can light coconut milk, shaken well

1 (15-ounce) can black beans, drained and rinsed

4 tablespoons tomato paste

1 tablespoon Thai red curry paste

Juice of 2 medium limes

1½ teaspoons ground cumin

1½ teaspoons ground paprika

¼ teaspoon ground allspice

¼ teaspoon freshly ground black pepper

1. Heat olive oil in a large stockpot over medium heat. Add onion, garlic, carrots, celery, bell pepper, and sweet potatoes and cook, stirring, 3 minutes, until they begin to sweat.

2. Add remaining ingredients and stir well to combine. Cover and simmer over medium heat, stirring frequently, 10 minutes.

3. Reduce heat to medium-low to low and simmer covered, stirring frequently, 5–10 minutes until sweet potatoes are fork tender. Keep checking to make sure the mixture isn't cooking too fast or beginning to stick and burn; lower heat if necessary.

4. Remove from heat and serve immediately.

PER SERVING Calories: 177 | Fat: 5.1 g | Protein: 7.4 g | Sodium: 262 mg | Fiber: 9.3 g | Carbohydrates: 26.8 g | Sugar: 6.9 g

Mexican Brown Rice and Beans

A super healthy recipe for rice and beans, you can enjoy this dish as a yummy side, or use it as a filling for burritos, tacos, nachos, and more. Stir in sautéed bell pepper, corn, tender sweet potato, diced avocado, and more for a complete one-dish meal.

PREP TIME: 5 minutes
COOK TIME: 45 minutes

INGREDIENTS | SERVES 4

1 tablespoon olive oil

1 teaspoon ground cumin

2 teaspoons chili seasoning

1 medium red onion, peeled and diced finely

1 cup uncooked brown rice, rinsed well

2 cups vegetable broth

1 tablespoon tomato paste

2 (15-ounce) cans pinto beans, drained and rinsed

¼ teaspoon freshly ground black pepper

¼ cup chopped fresh cilantro

1. Heat oil in a medium saucepan over medium heat. Add cumin and chili seasoning and sauté until fragrant, 30 seconds. Add onion and cook, stirring, 2 minutes, until it begins to sweat.

2. Add rice and stir well to coat. Add vegetable broth and tomato paste and combine. Bring to a boil over high heat, reduce heat to low, cover, and simmer until all of the liquid is absorbed, about 40 minutes.

3. Remove pan from heat and place contents in a large serving bowl. Add beans, pepper, and cilantro to rice mixture and stir to combine. Serve immediately.

PER SERVING Calories: 313 | Fat: 5.0 g | Protein: 9.6 g | Sodium: 719 mg | Fiber: 6.3 g | Carbohydrates: 57.4 g | Sugar: 3.2 g

Red Lentil Curry with Green Beans and Butternut Squash

This delicious dish gives you a sweet and savory curry filled with healthy plant protein and fiber. Precubed butternut squash is sold frozen at many supermarkets and if thawed can be used in this recipe; it's not only easy but inexpensive, too. Thawed frozen green beans may also be used instead of fresh. Serve plain or spoon over cooked brown rice, quinoa, or another favorite whole grain.

PREP TIME: 10 minutes
COOK TIME: 22 minutes

INGREDIENTS | SERVES 4

1 tablespoon olive oil

1 medium onion, peeled and diced

2 cups cubed butternut squash

1 tablespoon curry powder

1 teaspoon ground cumin

½ teaspoon dried red pepper flakes

⅛ teaspoon ground cloves

3 cups vegetable broth

1 cup uncooked red lentils

2 ripe medium tomatoes, diced

1 cup green beans, cut into 2" pieces

¾ cup light coconut milk

¼ cup chopped fresh cilantro

1. Heat oil in a medium stockpot over medium heat. Add onion and squash and cook, stirring, 4 minutes. Add curry powder, cumin, red pepper flakes, and cloves and stir until fragrant, 1 minute.

2. Reduce heat to medium-low. Stir in broth and lentils, cover, and simmer 10–12 minutes, stirring occasionally.

3. Uncover pot and add tomatoes, beans, and coconut milk. Cook uncovered until tomatoes and beans are tender, about 5 minutes.

4. Remove from heat and stir in cilantro. Serve immediately.

PER SERVING Calories: 305 | Fat: 7.3 g | Protein: 13.8 g | Sodium: 720 mg | Fiber: 9.6 g | Carbohydrates: 49.0 g | Sugar: 5.8 g

Whipped Butternut Squash

If you have any leftover butternut squash, use it in a delicious side dish! Puréed squash is a favorite recipe in New England and is super easy to make. Place cubed squash in a microwave-safe bowl, add ¼ cup water, and cover with plastic wrap. Microwave on high 10 minutes. Transfer contents to a food processor, add a tablespoon of broth, and purée. Season to taste.

Pasta with Chickpea and Tomato Sauce

This mock Bolognese sauce made from chopped chickpeas, onion, and seasoned tomatoes may become a family favorite. Healthy, inexpensive, and tasty, it elevates the humble bean to greater heights. Serve with your favorite whole-grain pasta; shells are particularly nice at holding the sauce for each bite.

PREP TIME: 15 minutes
COOK TIME: 30 minutes

INGREDIENTS | SERVES 6

1 (15-ounce) can chickpeas, drained and rinsed

2 teaspoons olive oil

1 large onion, peeled and chopped

1 medium carrot, peeled and minced

3 cloves garlic, minced

3 tablespoons red wine

1 teaspoon dried oregano

½ teaspoon dried basil

½ teaspoon dried thyme

½ teaspoon garlic powder

½ teaspoon ground paprika

¼ teaspoon freshly ground black pepper

⅛ teaspoon dried red pepper flakes

1 (28-ounce) can crushed tomatoes

1 tablespoon low-sodium soy sauce

1 tablespoon agave nectar

1 (12-ounce) package whole-grain pasta

3 tablespoons chopped fresh basil

3 tablespoons nutritional yeast

1. Place chickpeas in a food processor and pulse once or twice to chop coarsely. Set aside.

2. Heat oil in a medium sauté pan over medium heat. Add onion and carrot and cook, stirring, 3 minutes. Add garlic and sauté 2 minutes. Add chickpeas, red wine, oregano, dried basil, thyme, garlic powder, paprika, black pepper, and red pepper flakes and cook, stirring, 5 minutes, until tender.

3. Stir in tomatoes, soy sauce, and agave and bring to a simmer. Lower the heat to medium-low to low, cover, and simmer 20 minutes.

4. Cook pasta according to package directions, then drain.

5. Spoon sauce over pasta and sprinkle with fresh basil and nutritional yeast. Serve immediately.

PER SERVING Calories: 356 | Fat: 4.1 g | Protein: 14.0 g | Sodium: 441 mg | Fiber: 12.7 g | Carbohydrates: 68.1 g | Sugar: 13.3 g

Bean Salad with Orange Vinaigrette

Canned beans make this dish a snap to prepare; substitute 1½ cups of each type of cooked bean if you're making them yourself. Serve over your choice of leafy greens, either cooked or raw. Kidney beans may be substituted for one of the others if desired.

PREP TIME: 10 minutes
COOK TIME: N/A

INGREDIENTS | SERVES 6

1 (15-ounce) can black beans, drained and rinsed

1 (15-ounce) can chickpeas, drained and rinsed

1 (15-ounce) can pinto beans, drained and rinsed

1 small onion, peeled and chopped

1 medium carrot, peeled and shredded

1 medium bell pepper, seeded and diced

1 medium stalk celery, trimmed and diced

⅓ cup apple cider vinegar

¼ cup pure maple syrup

2 tablespoons orange juice

1 tablespoon olive oil

1 teaspoon grated orange zest

½ teaspoon freshly ground black pepper

1. Place beans in a large mixing bowl. Add onion, carrot, bell pepper, and celery and stir to combine.

2. Measure remaining ingredients into a small bowl and whisk well to combine. Pour dressing over salad and toss to coat.

3. Serve immediately or cover and refrigerate until serving.

PER SERVING Calories: 251 | Fat: 3.2 g | Protein: 12.0 g | Sodium: 304 mg | Fiber: 11.1 g | Carbohydrates: 43.6 g | Sugar: 13.0 g

Tasty Lentil Tacos

This recipe gives you a speedy and inexpensive MIND diet–appropriate meal the whole family will love. Cooked lentils are soft and brown, with a look and texture not unlike ground beef. Combined with sautéed onion, garlic, salsa, and seasoning, they make an amazing taco filling. This dish is absolutely warm, hearty, delicious, and so healthy. Substitute soft taco shells for the crunchy and a spicier salsa for the mild, if desired.

PREP TIME: 5 minutes
COOK TIME: 33 minutes

INGREDIENTS | SERVES 6

1 teaspoon olive oil
1 medium onion, peeled and diced
2 garlic cloves, minced
1 cup uncooked lentils, rinsed
1 tablespoon chili seasoning
2 teaspoons ground cumin
1 teaspoon dried oregano
2½ cups vegetable broth
1 (12 shell) package crunchy taco shells
1 cup mild salsa

1. Heat oil in a large skillet or sauté pan over medium heat. Add onion and garlic and cook, stirring, 3 minutes. Add the lentils, chili seasoning, cumin, and oregano and cook, stirring, 1 minute, until fragrant.

2. Add broth and bring to a boil over high heat; then reduce heat to low, cover, and simmer 30 minutes.

3. Warm taco shells according to directions on package.

4. Remove lentils from heat, uncover pan, and mash lentils slightly. Stir in salsa.

5. Spoon roughly ¼ cup filling into each taco shell and serve immediately.

PER SERVING Calories: 273 | Fat: 6.3 g | Protein: 10.7 g | Sodium: 836 mg | Fiber: 6.6 g | Carbohydrates: 43.8 g | Sugar: 4.4 g

Edamame with Corn and Cranberries

A delightfully chewy, crisp, and colorful way to brighten plates and palates year-round, this super-quick side is especially great for summer picnics and can be doubled or tripled to feed a crowd. Either freshly cooked corn or frozen thawed corn kernels may be used in this recipe. Dried cherries may be substituted for the cranberries if desired.

PREP TIME: 5 minutes
COOK TIME: N/A

INGREDIENTS | SERVES 4

1¼ cups shelled edamame

¾ cup corn kernels

1 small red pepper, seeded and diced

¼ cup dried sweetened cranberries

1 medium shallot, peeled and finely diced

2 tablespoons red wine vinegar

1 tablespoon olive oil

1 teaspoon agave nectar

1 teaspoon mustard

¼ teaspoon freshly ground black pepper

1. Place edamame, corn, bell pepper, cranberries, and shallot in a medium mixing bowl and stir to combine.

2. Measure remaining ingredients into a small bowl and whisk well.

3. Pour dressing over salad and toss well to coat.

4. Serve immediately or cover and refrigerate until serving.

PER SERVING Calories: 149 | Fat: 5.7 g | Protein: 6.5 g | Sodium: 21 mg | Fiber: 4.1 g | Carbohydrates: 19.2 g | Sugar: 9.8 g

Speedy Chana Masala

In this healthy and delicious version of the traditional Indian dish, chickpeas, tomatoes, and greens are simmered in a spicy, seasoned sauce. Serve this Speedy Chana Masala over cooked brown rice for a super satisfying meal. Swiss chard, baby kale, or spinach may be substituted for the collard greens if desired.

PREP TIME: 10 minutes
COOK TIME: 30 minutes

INGREDIENTS | SERVES 4

1½ cups vegetable broth, divided

1 medium onion, peeled and diced

3 cloves garlic, minced

1 fresh jalapeño pepper, seeded and minced

1 teaspoon curry powder

½ teaspoon garam masala

¼ teaspoon ground ginger

1 (15-ounce) can no salt added diced tomatoes, with juice

2 (15-ounce) cans chickpeas, drained and rinsed

4 cups chopped fresh collard greens, stems removed

¼ cup chopped fresh cilantro

1 tablespoon lemon juice

1. Heat ½ cup broth in a large sauté pan over medium-high heat. Add onion, garlic, and jalapeño and cook, stirring, 5 minutes.

2. Add curry powder, garam masala, and ginger and stir until fragrant. Add tomatoes, chickpeas, and remaining broth and bring to a simmer. Reduce heat to medium and cook, stirring frequently, 15 minutes.

3. Add collard greens, cover, and cook until tender, stirring occasionally, 10 minutes.

4. Remove from heat. Add cilantro and lemon juice and stir to combine. Serve immediately.

PER SERVING Calories: 225 | Fat: 2.3 g | Protein: 11.4 g | Sodium: 670 mg | Fiber: 11.9 g | Carbohydrates: 40.5 g | Sugar: 10.4 g

What Is Garam Masala?

Garam masala is a ground spice blend used extensively in Indian cooking. Though blends may differ, garam masala typically includes cinnamon, cumin, coriander, cloves, ginger, nutmeg, pepper, mace, star anise, and bay leaves. Garam masala is potent in terms of fragrance and flavor, but unlike many curry powders does not tend to be fiery hot.

Cilantro-Lime Black Bean Spread

Completely guilt-free and oh so good, this bean spread is made up of a chorus line of black beans, fresh cilantro, and garlic with a zippy lime high kick. Spread in sandwiches or serve with fresh vegetables and tortilla chips.

PREP TIME: 5 minutes
COOK TIME: N/A

INGREDIENTS | YIELDS 1½ CUPS

1 (15-ounce) can black beans, drained and rinsed

¼ cup fresh cilantro

2 cloves garlic

Juice of 1 medium lime

1½ teaspoons ground cumin

½ teaspoon ground coriander

¼ teaspoon chili seasoning

¼ teaspoon freshly ground black pepper

⅛ teaspoon ground cayenne

1. Place all ingredients in a food processor and pulse until smooth.

2. Serve immediately or cover and refrigerate until serving.

PER ¼-CUP SERVING Calories: 69 | Fat: 0.1 g | Protein: 5.3 g | Sodium: 97 mg | Fiber: 5.2 g | Carbohydrates: 12.3 g | Sugar: 1.3 g

Hot Tamale Pie

A hearty Southwestern filling of pinto beans, onion, garlic, and bell pepper baked beneath a blanketing crust of cornbread, this dish is absolutely delicious, not to mention healthy, easy, and inexpensive. Serve with sautéed collard greens and sliced watermelon for a fully balanced meal.

PREP TIME: 10 minutes
COOK TIME: 35 minutes

INGREDIENTS | SERVES 8

Olive oil cooking spray
1 teaspoon plus 2 tablespoons olive oil, divided
1 medium onion, peeled and diced
4 cloves garlic, minced
1 medium bell pepper, seeded and diced
¾ cup fresh or frozen corn kernels
2 (15-ounce) cans pinto beans, drained and rinsed
1 cup pasta sauce
1 teaspoon ground cumin
1 teaspoon chili seasoning
⅔ cup cornmeal
⅔ cup white whole-wheat flour
1 teaspoon baking powder
¾ cup almond milk
2 tablespoons agave nectar

1. Preheat oven to 350°F. Spray a deep-dish pie pan lightly with cooking spray and set aside.

2. Heat 1 teaspoon oil in a large sauté pan. Add onion and garlic and sauté 2 minutes. Add bell pepper, corn, beans, pasta sauce, cumin, and chili seasoning and sauté 2–3 minutes more. Remove from heat and transfer filling to the prepared pie pan. Set aside.

3. Measure cornmeal, flour, and baking powder into a medium mixing bowl and whisk to combine. Add milk, remaining 2 tablespoons oil, and agave and stir well to combine. Pour batter over filling in the pie pan and smooth to even.

4. Place pan on middle rack in oven and bake until golden brown, 30 minutes.

5. Remove from oven and serve immediately.

PER SERVING Calories: 287 | Fat: 6.2 g | Protein: 10.0 g | Sodium: 393 mg | Fiber: 8.6 g | Carbohydrates: 49.6 g | Sugar: 8.7 g

Focus on Plant-Based Meals

A vegan diet might sound crippling in its limitation, but in truth it's a liberating way of looking at food. Without meat on the menu, your focus broadens to include a far more diverse array of foods, and in far greater quantities, than before. Whether you're eating a plant-based diet all of the time or just occasionally, your body will thank you for it. Scientific studies have proven the long-term benefits to health of a diet rich in vegetables, fruit, and whole grains.

Roasted Chickpeas and Asparagus

A very simple side with a ton of delicious flavor, in this dish the chickpeas and fresh asparagus are tossed with a drizzle of sweet and salty dressing, then hot roasted. The result is a tender marriage of greens and protein you won't be able to stop devouring!

PREP TIME: 5 minutes
COOK TIME: 20 minutes

INGREDIENTS | SERVES 4

1 (15-ounce) can chickpeas, drained and rinsed

1 pound fresh asparagus, cut into 2" pieces

2 teaspoons sesame oil

1 teaspoon low-sodium soy sauce

1 teaspoon natural (unflavored) rice wine vinegar

1 teaspoon agave nectar

¼ teaspoon freshly ground black pepper

1. Preheat oven to 425°F. Line a baking sheet with parchment and set aside.

2. Place chickpeas and asparagus in a medium mixing bowl. Add remaining ingredients and toss well to coat.

3. Place baking sheet on middle rack in oven and bake 20 minutes, until tender.

4. Remove from oven and serve immediately.

PER SERVING Calories: 135 | Fat: 3.3 g | Protein: 7.1 g | Sodium: 177 mg | Fiber: 6.5 g | Carbohydrates: 20.4 g | Sugar: 5.9 g

Hearty Homemade Veggie Burgers

These homemade patties are healthy, filling, delectably moist, and absolutely delicious. The recipe yields 10 "beefy"-sized burgers, so there's plenty to enjoy. The recipe requires an investment of time (most of it hands-off), but these burgers freeze beautifully, so feel free to double the recipe and freeze for later meals.

PREP TIME: 1 hour 25 minutes
COOK TIME: 50 minutes

INGREDIENTS | SERVES 10

1½ cups uncooked lentils

4½ cups plus 6 tablespoons water, divided

2 tablespoons ground flaxseed

1 teaspoon olive oil

1 medium onion, peeled and chopped

2 cloves garlic, minced

4 ounces fresh mushrooms, chopped

1 medium stalk celery, trimmed and chopped

1 medium carrot, peeled and chopped

1 small bell pepper, seeded and chopped

1 cup chopped walnuts

1 teaspoon chili seasoning

½ teaspoon all-purpose seasoning

½ teaspoon ground cumin

½ teaspoon ground mustard

¼ teaspoon freshly ground black pepper

5 tablespoons tomato paste

½ cup quick oats

1. Rinse lentils well and place in a large saucepan; add 4½ cups water. Place pot over high heat and bring to a boil; then reduce heat to medium-low, cover pot, and simmer 25 minutes until lentils are tender but not mushy. Drain and set aside.

2. Line a large baking sheet with parchment and set aside.

3. Place flaxseed and 6 tablespoons water in a small bowl and whisk well to combine. Set aside to thicken.

4. Heat oil in a large sauté pan over medium heat. Add onion, garlic, mushrooms, celery, carrot, bell pepper, and walnuts and cook, stirring, 5 minutes.

5. Remove pan from heat and transfer contents to a large mixing bowl. Add lentils, flaxseed mixture, chili seasoning, all-purpose seasoning, cumin, mustard, black pepper, tomato paste, and oats and mix well. The mixture should be fairly solid.

6. Scoop mixture out using a ½-cup measuring cup and shape into patties. The burger mixture will be soft and a bit sticky, so scoop, pat, and form quickly. Place formed burgers on the parchment-lined baking sheet and refrigerate 1 hour.

continued on next page

7. To bake, position an oven rack in the top third of the oven. Preheat oven to 450°F. Place baking sheet on top rack in oven and bake 10 minutes. Remove sheet from oven and very gently flip burgers; they will be soft and delicate. Return to top rack in oven and bake 10 minutes, until lightly browned.

8. Remove baking sheet from oven, rest burgers 10 minutes, then serve. The burgers are very firm when cool, but while hot they're fragile so be careful.

9. Serve burgers warm or store in an airtight container and freeze for later consumption.

PER SERVING Calories: 222 | Fat: 8.9 g | Protein: 10.7 g | Sodium: 88 mg | Fiber: 5.6 g | Carbohydrates: 26.7 g | Sugar: 2.9 g

Kidney Beans with Carrots, Potatoes, and Kale

This hearty, one-pot meal is protein packed and filled with the earthy flavors of carrots, potatoes, and kale. The red wine adds a depth of flavor that's absolutely delicious. Serve over cooked brown rice for added heft. Spinach or collard greens may be substituted for the kale if desired.

PREP TIME: 10 minutes
COOK TIME: 30 minutes

INGREDIENTS | SERVES 4

1 tablespoon olive oil
1 medium onion, peeled and diced
3 cloves garlic, minced
3 medium carrots, peeled and diced
2 medium stalks celery, trimmed and diced
2 medium potatoes, peeled and diced
2½ cups vegetable broth
½ cup red wine
1¼ teaspoons ground cumin
1 teaspoon all-purpose seasoning
½ teaspoon ground coriander
½ teaspoon dried oregano
¼ teaspoon dried thyme
¼ teaspoon freshly ground black pepper
6 cups chopped fresh kale leaves
1 (15-ounce) can kidney beans, drained and rinsed
2 tablespoons lemon juice

1. Heat oil in a medium stockpot over medium heat. Add onion, garlic, carrots, and celery and cook, stirring, 5 minutes. Add potatoes, broth, wine, cumin, seasoning, coriander, oregano, thyme, and pepper and stir well to combine.

2. Bring to a boil over high heat, reduce heat to medium-low, cover pot, and simmer 15 minutes, stirring occasionally.

3. Uncover pot, add kale and beans, and stir to combine. Cover and simmer 10 minutes until kale is tender.

4. Remove from heat and stir in lemon juice. Serve immediately.

PER SERVING Calories: 264 | Fat: 4.3 g | Protein: 10.0 g | Sodium: 795 mg | Fiber: 9.6 g | Carbohydrates: 43.9 g | Sugar: 6.2 g

Instant Refried Beans

This fat-free, cholesterol-free, and incredibly tasty recipe comes together so fast, you can enjoy it anytime the craving hits. Roll it up in tortillas with sautéed onion, peppers, and salsa or use as a spread for crackers and raw vegetables. Swap kidney or black beans for the pinto.

PREP TIME: 2 minutes
COOK TIME: N/A

INGREDIENTS | SERVES 3

1 (15-ounce) can pinto beans
1 teaspoon onion powder
½ teaspoon garlic powder
¼ teaspoon ground cumin
¼ teaspoon low-sodium soy sauce
¼ teaspoon freshly ground black pepper

1. Drain beans, reserve the liquid, and rinse well.

2. Place beans, onion powder, garlic powder, cumin, soy sauce, and pepper in a food processor and pulse until smooth; add ¼ cup of the reserved bean liquid to thin if desired.

3. Serve immediately.

PER SERVING Calories: 121 | Fat: 0.5 g | Protein: 7.4 g | Sodium: 230 mg | Fiber: 5.4 g | Carbohydrates: 22.1 g | Sugar: 0.8 g

Pinto Bean Facts

Pinto in Spanish means "painted," which describes the speckled exterior of these tasty and nutritious beans. High in protein, folate, fiber, and minerals, pinto beans are an excellent addition to a healthy diet. Add them to chilies, soups, and salads; layer with vegetables and bake for a hot casserole; or mash to make a dip or sandwich spread.

Brown Rice with Mango, Black Beans, and Lime

This easy side is a fabulous way to reuse leftover rice. Delicious warm or cold, it showcases the simple, fresh flavors the best way possible: naked! If you don't have a ripe mango, substitute 1½ cups diced pineapple.

PREP TIME: 10 minutes
COOK TIME: N/A

INGREDIENTS | SERVES 6

3 cups cooked brown rice

1 (15-ounce) can black beans, drained and rinsed

1 ripe mango, peeled, cored, and diced

1 medium red bell pepper, seeded and diced

2 scallions, sliced

2 cloves garlic, minced

Juice of 2 medium limes

¼ cup chopped fresh cilantro

¼ teaspoon freshly ground black pepper

1. Place all ingredients in a large mixing bowl and stir well to combine.

2. Serve immediately or cover and refrigerate until serving.

PER SERVING Calories: 216 | Fat: 0.9 g | Protein: 8.1 g | Sodium: 94 mg | Fiber: 8.2 g | Carbohydrates: 44.8 g | Sugar: 9.7 g

Barbecued Tempeh

A marvelous take on vegan sloppy joes, this tangy Barbecued Tempeh makes a quick and tasty meal, and is as filling as it is flavorful. Serve in buns or spoon over your choice of cooked brown rice, whole-grain pasta, quinoa, couscous, baked potatoes, or sweet potatoes.

PREP TIME: 10 minutes
COOK TIME: 20 minutes
INGREDIENTS | SERVES 6

2 teaspoons olive oil

1 (8-ounce) package organic tempeh, diced

1 large onion, peeled and diced

1 medium bell pepper, seeded and diced

3 cloves garlic, minced

1 (15-ounce) can no salt added diced tomatoes

2 (8-ounce) can tomato sauce

1 tablespoon apple cider vinegar

1 tablespoon molasses

1½ teaspoons Worcestershire sauce

1 teaspoon ground paprika

½ teaspoon freshly ground black pepper

½ teaspoon ground cumin

¼ teaspoon ground cinnamon

¼ teaspoon liquid smoke

⅛ teaspoon ground cayenne

¼ cup chopped fresh cilantro

1. Heat oil in a medium sauté pan over medium heat. Add tempeh, onion, bell pepper, and garlic and sauté for 5 minutes.

2. Add tomatoes, tomato sauce, vinegar, molasses, Worcestershire sauce, paprika, black pepper, cumin, cinnamon, liquid smoke, and cayenne. Reduce heat to medium-low and cook 15 minutes, stirring frequently.

3. Remove from heat and stir in cilantro. Serve immediately.

PER SERVING Calories: 145 | Fat: 5.2 g | Protein: 9.1 g | Sodium: 406 mg | Fiber: 3.2 g | Carbohydrates: 17.6 g | Sugar: 9.0 g

What Is Tempeh?

Tempeh is a fermented soybean product sold in firm, rectangular cakes. It has a rugged texture and nutty flavor that melds well with many types of food. Cut it into cubes and add to pasta sauce, sauté along with vegetables, or marinate in your favorite sauce and bake. Tempeh is cholesterol-free and a good source of protein, calcium, and iron. Look for it in the grocery store produce section; it's typically stocked in the refrigerated case alongside the tofu.

Spicy Chickpea Tacos with Arugula

These Spicy Chickpea Tacos with Arugula are just about the tastiest tacos ever! They are coated with a thick and spicy tomato-based sauce dotted with chickpeas, the peppery cool of arugula, and the crunchy bite of corn. Feel free to spoon any extra filling over tortilla chips or cooked brown rice if you run short of shells. For spicier tacos, increase the amount of pepper and pepper flakes.

PREP TIME: 10 minutes
COOK TIME: 10 minutes

INGREDIENTS | SERVES 6

1 (12 shell) package taco shells

2 (15-ounce) cans chickpeas, drained and rinsed

4 tablespoons tomato paste

1 tablespoon apple cider vinegar

1 tablespoon brown sugar

2 teaspoons chili seasoning

1 teaspoon ground mustard

1 teaspoon onion powder

½ teaspoon garlic powder

¼ teaspoon freshly ground black pepper

⅛ teaspoon dried red pepper flakes

6 cups fresh arugula, washed and dried

1. Heat taco shells according to package directions.

2. Add remaining ingredients except arugula to a large saucepan and stir well to combine.

3. Place pan over medium heat and simmer, stirring frequently, 10 minutes.

4. Remove pan from heat. Fill warm taco shells with arugula and then spoon chickpea mixture over top. Serve immediately.

PER SERVING Calories: 265 | Fat: 6.7 g | Protein: 8.9 g | Sodium: 387 mg | Fiber: 8.1 g | Carbohydrates: 41.1 g | Sugar: 7.1 g

Poultry

Red Wine Roasted Chicken

With delectably juicy chicken, infused with the richness of red wine and herbs, this recipe is guaranteed to become a new favorite. Make the marinade first thing in the morning and allow the bird to marinate until midafternoon to absorb maximum flavor. Baste several times throughout cooking to ensure moist, tender meat. Partner with roasted potatoes and steamed broccoli for a holiday-worthy meal anytime.

PREP TIME: 6 hours
COOK TIME: 1 hour 25 minutes
INGREDIENTS | SERVES 6

1 cup red wine
3 tablespoons olive oil
2 tablespoons balsamic vinegar
3 cloves garlic, minced
1 teaspoon dried thyme
1 teaspoon dried marjoram
½ teaspoon dried basil
½ teaspoon dried rosemary, crushed
½ teaspoon ground mustard
½ teaspoon ground sage
¼ teaspoon freshly ground black pepper[
1 (4-pound) whole chicken

1. Measure wine, oil, vinegar, garlic, thyme, marjoram, basil, rosemary, mustard, sage, and pepper into a large gallon-sized zip-top bag; seal and shake well to combine. Place chicken in the bag and make sure the seal is secure. Shake well, then place in refrigerator and marinate 6 hours.

2. Preheat oven to 450°F. Remove bird from marinade bag and place breast-side down in a small roaster pan. Pour marinade into pan. Place pan on middle rack in oven and roast 25 minutes.

3. Remove pan from oven. Reduce heat to 350°F. Gently flip bird breast-side up. Return pan to middle rack in oven and roast an additional 45–60 minutes; baste occasionally until chicken reaches an internal temperature of 165°F.

4. Remove pan from oven, rest chicken at least 15 minutes, then carve and serve immediately.

PER SERVING Calories: 542 | Fat: 32.2 g | Protein: 51.0 g | Sodium: 155 mg | Fiber: 0.3 g | Carbohydrates: 1.8 g | Sugar: 0.9 g

Lemon-Herb Roasted Chicken

If you crave those super-aromatic lemony roasted chickens sold at many supermarkets, then get ready to fall in love. Delicately flavored with fresh citrus and herbs, this deliciously roasted chicken will leave you and your lucky dinner companions happy and healthy.

PREP TIME: 10 minutes
COOK TIME: 1 hour

INGREDIENTS | SERVES 6

1 teaspoon plus 1 tablespoon olive oil, divided

1½ teaspoons dried thyme

½ teaspoon, dried basil

½ teaspoon freshly ground black pepper

1 (4-pound) whole chicken

3 garlic cloves, minced

1 medium lemon, cut into wedges

1 bay leaf

1 small onion, peeled and quartered

½ cup dry white wine

½ teaspoon all-purpose seasoning

1. Preheat oven to 350°F. Lightly oil a small roasting pan with 1 teaspoon olive oil and set aside.

2. Combine thyme, basil, and pepper in a small bowl. Set aside.

3. Brush the outside of the bird with 1 tablespoon olive oil, then sprinkle with herb mixture.

4. Place chicken breast-side up in the roasting pan. Put garlic, lemon wedges, bay leaf, and onion inside the chicken. Pour wine into the pan. Sprinkle the outside of the chicken with seasoning.

5. Place the pan on the middle rack in the oven and bake roughly 1 hour, until chicken reaches an internal temperature of 165°F and juices run clear when a thigh is pierced with a sharp knife.

6. Remove from oven, rest bird 15 minutes, then carve and serve immediately.

PER SERVING Calories: 515 | Fat: 27.8 g | Protein: 51.0 g | Sodium: 155 mg | Fiber: 0.4 g | Carbohydrates: 2.3 g | Sugar: 0.7 g

One-Pot Chicken and Vegetables

For this dish meaty chicken breasts are first breaded in a seasoned flour, then browned to a golden crisp, so they retain their shape and yummy coating during cooking rather than simply falling apart like a stew. The tender-crisp vegetables and herb-flecked broth bathe the succulent breaded breasts, resulting in a sensational "best of both worlds" one-pot meal.

PREP TIME: 10–15 minutes
COOK TIME: 45–60 minutes

INGREDIENTS | SERVES 4

1 cup white whole-wheat flour

1½ teaspoons freshly ground black pepper, divided

1 teaspoon garlic powder

1 teaspoon ground paprika

4 (4-ounce) boneless, skinless chicken breasts

3 tablespoons olive oil

1 medium onion, peeled and chopped

3 cloves garlic, minced

3 medium stalks celery, trimmed and chopped

5 medium carrots, peeled and cut into 1" pieces

6 small potatoes, halved or quartered

1 tablespoon herbes de Provence

½ teaspoon dried rosemary, crushed

1½ cups chicken broth

Herbes de Provence

A classic blend of French herbs, typically composed of dried basil, thyme, savory, fennel, and lavender, herbes de Provence gives a distinct flavor to many dishes and is particularly well suited to fowl and seafood. Commercial blends are sold in many supermarkets and online.

1. Preheat oven to 375°F. Get out a lidded Dutch oven (or similar ovensafe pot) and set aside.

2. Measure flour into a medium mixing bowl. Add 1 teaspoon pepper, garlic powder, and paprika and whisk well to combine. Dredge chicken breasts in seasoned flour, coating each thoroughly.

3. Heat oil in the Dutch oven over medium heat until it simmers. Add breasts two at a time to hot oil and fry just until the outside is golden brown, about 2 minutes per side. Remove from pot, place on towel to drain, and repeat with other two breasts. Set aside.

4. Add onion, garlic, and celery to the (now empty) pot. Cook, stirring, 5 minutes, then add carrots and potatoes and stir to combine.

5. Place browned chicken breasts on top, then sprinkle with herbes de Provence, rosemary, and ½ teaspoon pepper. Pour broth over top and cover with lid. Place on the middle rack in the oven and bake covered 30–45 minutes until carrots and potatoes are soft.

6. Remove from oven and plate each chicken breast with ¼ of the vegetables and ¼ of the broth. Serve immediately.

PER SERVING Calories: 479 | Fat: 8.9 g | Protein: 33.7 g | Sodium: 434 mg | Fiber: 9.3 g | Carbohydrates: 68.0 g | Sugar: 6.9 g

Slow Cooker Chicken with Butternut Squash and Kale

This healthy and flavorful one-dish meal is delicious as is, but it's even better served over cooked whole-grain couscous, brown rice, or quinoa. If pressed for time, butternut squash is often sold in precubed packages; you will need roughly 1½ pounds for this recipe. For variety, substitute cubed sweet potatoes for the butternut squash, collard greens or Swiss chard for the kale, and kidney or black beans for the chickpeas. Before serving, sprinkle with chopped almonds or walnuts for added protein and crunch.

PREP TIME: 15 minutes
COOK TIME: 4–8 hours

INGREDIENTS | SERVES 8

1 medium butternut squash (about 1½ pounds), halved, seeded, peeled, and cut into 2" cubes

2 pounds boneless, skinless chicken thighs, cut into large pieces

4 cups chopped fresh kale leaves

2 (15-ounce) cans no salt added diced tomatoes, with juice

1 large onion, peeled and diced

3 cloves garlic, minced

1 (15-ounce) can chickpeas, drained and rinsed

¼ cup seedless raisins

1 cup chicken broth

1 tablespoon apple cider vinegar

1 tablespoon agave nectar

1 tablespoon ground cumin

2 teaspoons ground coriander

1 teaspoon all-purpose seasoning

½ teaspoon ground cinnamon

½ teaspoon ground ginger

½ teaspoon freshly ground black pepper

1. Add all ingredients to a slow cooker and stir to combine.

2. Cover slow cooker and cook on low 7–8 hours or on high 4–5 hours, stirring occasionally if possible. Serve hot.

PER SERVING Calories: 267 | Fat: 4.1 g | Protein: 26.8 g | Sodium: 410 mg | Fiber: 6.7 g | Carbohydrates: 31.5 g | Sugar: 12.1 g

Herbed Chicken Paprikash

This flavorful version of the traditional Hungarian dish uses dried herbs instead of salt and substitutes nonfat yogurt for sour cream. Spinach, mushrooms, and carrots boost the nutritional profile, making this a healthier, more colorful meal that's perfect for those following the MIND diet.

PREP TIME: 10 minutes
COOK TIME: 35 minutes

INGREDIENTS | SERVES 4

½ teaspoon dried oregano

¼ teaspoon dried thyme

¼ teaspoon dried basil

⅛ teaspoon dried rosemary

4 (8-ounce) chicken leg quarters, skin removed

1 teaspoon olive oil

⅓ cup dry white wine

⅓ cup chicken broth

1 small onion, peeled and sliced thinly

⅔ cup sliced fresh button mushrooms

¼ cup finely grated carrots

4 cups chopped fresh baby spinach

2 tablespoons white whole-wheat flour

2 tablespoons water

2 teaspoons ground paprika

2 tablespoons plain nonfat yogurt

The Beauty of Paprika

Paprika is a powdered seasoning made from ground chili peppers, prized for both its flavor and its beautiful bright red color. Paprika is sold in both hot and sweet varieties. All of the recipes in this book call for the mild (sweet) version. Although it's often associated with Hungarian cuisine, paprika originated in the New World, in Mexico, and traveled east to Spain and Europe in the sixteenth century.

1. Measure oregano, thyme, basil, and rosemary into a small bowl and stir to combine.

2. Heat a large nonstick skillet over medium heat. Brush both sides of the chicken with oil and sprinkle evenly with herb mixture. Add chicken to the skillet and cook on both sides until browned, roughly 2 minutes per side.

3. Add wine and chicken broth to pan and bring to a boil. Reduce heat, cover, and simmer 20 minutes. Add onion, mushrooms, and carrots; cover and simmer 8 minutes. Add spinach and cook 2 minutes more. Remove chicken from pan and place on serving plate. Cover to keep warm.

4. Mix together flour and water in a small bowl; whisk to remove any lumps. Add mixture to the pan and increase heat to medium; bring to a boil and stir constantly. Cook over medium heat and stir until mixture thickens.

5. Stir in paprika. Remove from heat and stir in yogurt. Pour sauce over chicken. Serve immediately.

PER SERVING Calories: 135 | Fat: 3.4 g | Protein: 14.1 g | Sodium: 161 mg | Fiber: 2.3 g | Carbohydrates: 8.5 g | Sugar: 2.3 g

Chicken Cacciatore

This classic Italian dish is infused with the flavors of onion, garlic, red wine, and tomatoes. The chicken is first pan-seared to seal in its juices, then slowly simmered in the sauce. Sprinkle with grated Parmesan cheese before serving or pair with pasta and a green salad for an authentic Mediterranean meal.

PREP TIME: 5 minutes
COOK TIME: 60 minutes

INGREDIENTS | SERVES 4

1 tablespoon olive oil

1 large onion, peeled and diced

4 (4-ounce) boneless, skinless chicken breasts

¼ teaspoon freshly ground black pepper

2 tablespoons dry red wine

1 (15-ounce) can tomato sauce

1 teaspoon garlic powder

1 teaspoon dried basil

½ teaspoon dried oregano

¼ teaspoon dried parsley

⅛ teaspoon ground mustard

⅛ teaspoon dried red pepper flakes

1 teaspoon lemon juice

1 teaspoon sugar

¼ cup grated Parmesan cheese

1. Heat a large nonstick skillet over medium heat. Add oil and onion; sauté 5 minutes, until tender. Push onion to the edges of the pan.

2. Add chicken breasts. Sprinkle black pepper over chicken. Pan-fry for 2 minutes on each side. Remove chicken from the pan and transfer to a bowl or platter; set aside.

3. Add wine to the pan. Bring to a boil and cook 2 minutes; use a spoon or spatula to stir well and scrape and deglaze the bottom of the pan.

4. Add tomato sauce, garlic powder, basil, oregano, parsley, mustard, red pepper flakes, lemon juice, and sugar to the pan; stir to combine.

5. Add chicken back to the pan and spoon some of the tomato sauce over the top of the chicken. Reduce heat to low, cover, and simmer 45 minutes. Remove pan from heat, top with Parmesan, and serve immediately.

PER SERVING Calories: 230 | Fat: 6.6 g | Protein: 27.7 g | Sodium: 618 mg | Fiber: 2.5 g | Carbohydrates: 12.2 g | Sugar: 6.5 g

Mustard-Maple Chicken with Potato Wedges

The mustard-maple marinade, a mix of maple syrup, mustard, olive oil, and apple cider vinegar, is used to marinate as well as to cook the chicken, resulting in a stupendously flavorful meal. Substitute other chicken parts for the boneless, skinless thighs if you so desire. Just be sure to cook until the meat is no longer pink when pierced and juices run clear.

PREP TIME: 2–3 hours
COOK TIME: 35–45 minutes

INGREDIENTS | SERVES 6

¼ cup pure maple syrup

2 tablespoons apple cider vinegar

2 tablespoons olive oil

2 tablespoons mustard

½ teaspoon freshly ground black pepper

2 pounds boneless, skinless chicken thighs

6 medium Yukon gold potatoes, scrubbed and cut into 8 wedges per potato

1½ teaspoons all-purpose seasoning

Don't Waste Oven Space

Oven-baked meals are super convenient, and even more so when you take advantage of extra oven space to simultaneously roast some vegetables. Let your cabinets and creativity be your guide. Cut broccoli into florets, halve Brussels sprouts, cube sweet or regular potatoes, trim green beans or asparagus, dice onion, and more. Add flavor by tossing the vegetables with all-purpose seasoning and freshly ground black pepper, a drizzle of olive oil, lemon juice, low-sodium soy sauce, or hot sauce. Arrange in a single layer on a parchment-lined baking sheet and place in the hot oven alongside the main dish. You'll have an absolutely delicious, highly nutritious side with little added effort.

1. Combine maple syrup, vinegar, oil, mustard, and pepper in a large gallon-sized zip-top bag. Seal and shake well to combine.

2. Add chicken to the marinade bag, seal, and invert several times to coat. Refrigerate 2–3 hours.

3. Preheat oven to 400°F. Oil a large 9" × 13" baking dish and set aside. Remove chicken from the refrigerator and set aside.

4. Place potatoes in a large mixing bowl, add seasoning, and toss well to coat.

5. Arrange potatoes in a single layer in the baking dish. Place dish on middle rack in oven and bake 15 minutes.

6. Remove from oven. Add chicken and marinade to the pan and return to the middle rack in the oven. Bake 20–30 minutes until potato wedges are tender and chicken has an internal temperature of 165°F and is no longer pink inside. Remove from oven and serve immediately.

PER SERVING Calories: 354 | Fat: 7.9 g | Protein: 32.8 g | Sodium: 302 mg | Fiber: 2.5 g | Carbohydrates: 36.3 g | Sugar: 5.1 g

Grilled Jerk Chicken

This Grilled Jerk Chicken gives you authentic Jamaican flavor, with MIND diet–approved flavors! Traditional Jamaican jerk seasoning relies heavily on fiery hot Scotch bonnet peppers; this milder version substitutes ground cayenne instead. The chicken is dry rubbed with a homemade jerk blend, then grilled on an indoor grill. Feel free to fire up the grill outside, or oven-bake the breasts at 400°F roughly 30 minutes until they reach an internal temperature of 165°F.

PREP TIME: 10 minutes
COOK TIME: 5 minutes

INGREDIENTS | SERVES 4

1 teaspoon Jerk Seasoning (see sidebar)
2 teaspoons fresh lime juice
1 teaspoon low-sodium soy sauce
1 teaspoon olive oil
1 medium jalapeño, seeded and chopped
2 scallions, white and green part chopped
1 teaspoon agave nectar
¼ teaspoon ground mustard
4 (4-ounce) boneless, skinless chicken breasts

1. Preheat a George Foreman–style indoor grill or heat a large grill pan over medium-high heat.

2. Add jerk seasoning, lime juice, soy sauce, oil, jalapeño, scallions, agave, and mustard to a small food processor and purée.

3. Rub both sides of chicken with spice mixture. Grill 3–5 minutes until chicken is cooked through and the juices run clear. Rest chicken 5 minutes, then serve.

PER SERVING Calories: 139 | Fat: 2.7 g | Protein: 24.4 g | Sodium: 41 mg | Fiber: 0.4 g | Carbohydrates: 2.4 g | Sugar: 1.6 g

Jerk Seasoning

To make your own jerk seasoning at home, combine the following: 1 tablespoon brown mustard seeds, 1 tablespoon onion powder, 2 teaspoons ground ginger, 2 teaspoons garlic powder, 1 teaspoon ground allspice, 1 teaspoon paprika, ½ teaspoon dried thyme, ½ teaspoon fennel seeds, ½ teaspoon black pepper, ½ teaspoon cayenne, and ¼ teaspoon ground cloves. Pulse in a small food processor until combined. Store excess in a sealed container in a cool, dark place; it will keep well for up to 2 years. This recipe yields a generous ⅓ cup of seasoning.

Oven-Baked Barbecue Chicken

Grilling not an option? Try this simple one-dish recipe instead. It's full of barbecue deliciousness and amazingly tender meat, but with all of the convenience of oven baking. Enjoy it as is, or cut the breasts into chunks before cooking and afterward spoon the chicken and sauce over whole-grain pasta, brown rice, quinoa, or baked potatoes. Substitute bone-in chicken if preferred; bake until the meat reaches an internal temperature of 165°F.

PREP TIME: 5 minutes
COOK TIME: 40 minutes

INGREDIENTS | SERVES 6

2½ pounds boneless, skinless chicken breasts

1 tablespoon olive oil

1 medium onion, peeled and diced

1 small green bell pepper, seeded and diced

1 medium stalk celery, trimmed and diced

3 cloves garlic, minced

2 (8-ounce) cans tomato sauce

2 tablespoons apple cider vinegar

1½ tablespoons molasses

1 tablespoon agave nectar

1 teaspoon liquid smoke

2 teaspoons ground cumin

2 teaspoons ground paprika

1 teaspoon dried oregano

1 teaspoon all-purpose seasoning

¼ teaspoon freshly ground black pepper

¼ teaspoon ground cayenne

1. Preheat oven to 400°F.

2. Arrange breasts in an ovenproof baking dish; set aside.

3. Heat oil in a medium saucepan over medium heat. Add onion, green pepper, and celery and cook, stirring, 3 minutes, until they begin to sweat. Add garlic and sauté 1–2 minutes more. Add remaining ingredients, reduce heat to medium-low, and simmer 5 minutes until bubbly, stirring frequently. Turn heat down if the sauce begins to bubble and pop out of the pot.

4. Remove sauce from heat and pour over chicken breasts. Cover the baking dish with a lid or aluminum foil and place on middle rack in oven. Bake until breasts are cooked through and no longer pink inside, about 30 minutes.

5. Remove baking dish from oven and serve immediately.

PER SERVING Calories: 281 | Fat: 5.1 g | Protein: 41.7 g | Sodium: 368 mg | Fiber: 2.4 g | Carbohydrates: 14.3 g | Sugar: 10.3 g

Chicken and Sweet Potato Stir-Fry

These seemingly incongruous elements make for one of the most deliciously different stir-fries around. Serve over cooked brown rice, quinoa, or mixed greens and top with chopped unsalted peanuts or cashews. Vegetable broth may be substituted for the chicken in a pinch.

PREP TIME: 10 minutes
COOK TIME: 18 minutes

INGREDIENTS | SERVES 4

1 tablespoon olive oil

2 medium sweet potatoes, peeled and cut into cut into 1" × 3" pieces

½ cup chicken broth

1 pound boneless, skinless chicken breasts

1 medium red onion, peeled and cut into 1" dice

¼ cup natural (unflavored) rice wine vinegar

3 tablespoons low-sodium soy sauce

6 scallions, sliced, whites and greens kept separate

1 cup frozen peas

2 cloves garlic, minced

½ teaspoon ground ginger

1 teaspoon sesame oil

1 tablespoon cornstarch

½ teaspoon freshly ground black pepper

1. Heat oil in a large skillet over medium-high heat until it simmers. Add sweet potatoes and stir to coat. Add broth and cover the pan. Cook, stirring occasionally, 10 minutes.

2. Remove the cover and add chicken, onion, vinegar, and soy sauce and stir well to combine. Cook uncovered 5 minutes, stirring occasionally.

3. Add scallion whites, frozen peas, garlic, ginger, and sesame oil and stir to combine. Cook 2 minutes, then add cornstarch. Stir well to coat. Cook 1 more minute to thicken the sauce, then remove from heat.

4. Garnish with scallion greens and pepper. Serve immediately.

PER SERVING Calories: 251 | Fat: 6.0 g | Protein: 28.5 g | Sodium: 546 mg | Fiber: 4.2 g | Carbohydrates: 18.4 g | Sugar: 4.8 g

Poultry Primer

A MIND diet healthy menu calls for smaller meat entrées. When you plan your meals to include lots of whole grains, vegetables, and fruit, 3–4 ounces of meat is usually a sufficient serving. As a general rule, a whole chicken breast is split in half to yield 2 servings. The cooked meat yield (minus the bones) will depend on the size of the breast, but is usually around 6 ounces per half breast, so a whole breast is sometimes enough for 4 servings. The cooked-meat yield for a chicken leg will be around 2 ounces; a thigh will yield 3–4 ounces, on average.

Kung Pao Chicken

The spicy bite of ginger, the tang of rice wine vinegar, the smoky depth of sesame oil, and that certain indescribable something that says "I am Chinese takeout" is all here in this MIND diet–friendly Kung Pao Chicken!

PREP TIME: 10 minutes
COOK TIME: 10 minutes

INGREDIENTS | SERVES 4

1 cup chicken broth

2 tablespoons low-sodium soy sauce

1 tablespoon balsamic vinegar

5 tablespoons cornstarch, divided

2 teaspoons sesame oil

1 teaspoon sugar

1 pound boneless, skinless chicken breasts, cubed

¼ teaspoon freshly ground black pepper

2 tablespoons olive oil, divided

¼ teaspoon dried red pepper flakes

2 tablespoons minced fresh ginger

6 scallions, sliced, whites and greens kept separate

1 medium red bell pepper, seeded and cubed

2 medium stalks celery, trimmed and sliced

2 medium carrots, peeled and sliced

¼ cup natural (unflavored) rice wine vinegar

¼ cup unsalted cashews, chopped

1. Place chicken broth, soy sauce, balsamic vinegar, 1 tablespoon cornstarch, sesame oil, and sugar in a small bowl. Whisk well to combine and set aside.

2. Place chicken in a medium mixing bowl, add 4 tablespoons cornstarch and black pepper, and toss well to coat using a pair of tongs.

3. Heat 1 tablespoon oil in a medium sauté pan over medium heat. Add chicken and cook until lightly browned on all sides, about 4 minutes total.

4. Add remaining 1 tablespoon oil to the pan. Add red pepper flakes, ginger, and scallion whites and cook, stirring, 1 minute.

5. Add bell pepper, celery, and carrots and sauté until they soften slightly, about 2 minutes.

6. Add rice vinegar and scrape the bottom of the pan to incorporate any browned bits.

7. Give chicken broth mixture a quick whisk, then add to the pan.

8. Check the chicken. If still pink inside, reduce heat and cook a couple minutes more. Remove pan from heat, sprinkle chicken with nuts and scallion greens, and serve immediately.

PER SERVING Calories: 315 | Fat: 13.6 g | Protein: 26.9 g | Sodium: 330 mg | Fiber: 1.8 g | Carbohydrates: 18.3 g | Sugar: 4.0 g

Spicy Sweet-and-Sour Chicken

If you adore Asian cooking, this is a must-try recipe. Here, spicy, sweet, and tangy bites of tender chicken are simmered with pineapple, onion, and green pepper in a flavorful sauce. Sriracha, which is a key ingredient, is a bottled red chili sauce sold in the international foods section of many supermarkets. If you can't find it, substitute an equal amount of hot sauce or dried red pepper flakes.

PREP TIME: 10 minutes
COOK TIME: 8 minutes

INGREDIENTS | SERVES 4

1 pound boneless, skinless chicken breasts, cut into 1" cubes

2 tablespoons cornstarch, divided

3 tablespoons low-sodium soy sauce, divided

1 (8-ounce) can pineapple chunks, in juice (liquid reserved)

¼ cup apple cider vinegar

¼ cup sugar

2 tablespoons ketchup

2 teaspoons sriracha

½ teaspoon ground ginger

1 tablespoon olive oil

1 small onion, peeled and diced

2 cloves garlic, minced

1 medium bell pepper, seeded and diced

1. Combine chicken, 1 tablespoon cornstarch, and 1 tablespoon soy sauce in a small bowl; toss well to coat. Set aside.

2. Drain liquid from the pineapple into another small bowl. Then measure in remaining 1 tablespoon cornstarch, remaining 2 tablespoons soy sauce, vinegar, sugar, ketchup, sriracha, and ginger; whisk to combine. Set aside.

3. Heat a large skillet over medium-high heat. Add oil and swirl to coat. Add chicken to pan and cook, stirring, 3 minutes. Add onion and garlic and sauté 1 minute. Stir in pineapple and bell pepper and cook, stirring, 3 minutes. Stir in sauce mixture and cook, stirring constantly, 1 minute. The vegetables should be tender and chicken should be cooked through and no longer pink inside.

4. Remove from heat and serve immediately.

PER SERVING Calories: 281 | Fat: 4.9 g | Protein: 25.9 g | Sodium: 502 mg | Fiber: 1.3 g | Carbohydrates: 31.9 g | Sugar: 24.6 g

Oven-Baked Chicken Tenders

Oven-baked, these crispy tenders are much lower in fat than their deep-fried counterparts, but have a whole lot of flavor. These freeze wonderfully; place leftovers into an airtight container for later meals. Serve with ketchup, barbecue sauce, and honey for dipping.

PREP TIME: 10 minutes
COOK TIME: 15 minutes

INGREDIENTS | SERVES 8

Olive oil cooking spray
½ cup unbleached all-purpose flour
½ cup white whole-wheat flour
½ cup bread crumbs
2 teaspoons garlic powder
2 teaspoons onion powder
1 teaspoon ground paprika
1 teaspoon freshly ground black pepper
½ cup skim milk
1 large egg white
3 pounds boneless, skinless chicken breast tenderloins

1. Preheat oven to 375°F. Take out a large baking sheet, cover with aluminum foil, spray lightly with cooking spray, and set aside.

2. Combine flours, bread crumbs, garlic powder, onion powder, paprika, and pepper in a large zip-top plastic bag. Seal and shake well to combine.

3. Whisk together milk and egg white in a shallow bowl.

4. One piece at a time, dip chicken into milk mixture, then place in flour bag, seal, and shake vigorously to coat. Place breaded tenders on the prepared baking sheet.

5. Place baking sheet on middle rack in oven and bake 10–15 minutes until golden brown.

6. Remove from oven and serve immediately.

PER SERVING Calories: 203 | Fat: 0.4 g | Protein: 36.0 g | Sodium: 313 mg | Fiber: 1.4 g | Carbohydrates: 13.2 g | Sugar: 0.4 g

Turkey Meatloaf

In this dish, ground turkey is flavored with a tangy herbed tomato sauce and sautéed vegetables, and sealed with a homey ketchup glaze. If you prefer, bake the loaf in a small, lightly oiled bread pan. If you don't have bread crumbs, make your own using the directions in the sidebar, or use an equal amount of rolled quick oats instead. Ground chicken may be substituted for the turkey if desired.

PREP TIME: 5 minutes
COOK TIME: 65 minutes

INGREDIENTS | SERVES 6

2 teaspoons olive oil, divided
1 medium onion, peeled and diced
2 medium stalks celery, trimmed and diced
1 medium green bell pepper, seeded and diced
1 medium carrot, peeled and shredded
6 cloves garlic, minced
1½ pounds lean ground turkey
1 (8-ounce) can tomato sauce
1 large egg
¾ cup bread crumbs
1 tablespoon molasses
1 tablespoon apple cider vinegar
2 teaspoons all-purpose seasoning
1 teaspoon dried basil
½ teaspoon dried oregano
½ teaspoon dried thyme
½ teaspoon ground mustard
½ teaspoon freshly ground black pepper
¼ cup ketchup

1. Preheat oven to 350°F. Lightly oil an 8" square baking pan with 1 teaspoon oil and set aside.

2. Heat 1 teaspoon oil in a nonstick skillet over medium heat. Add onion and cook, stirring, 2 minutes. Add celery, green pepper, carrot, and garlic and sauté 3 minutes. Remove from heat.

3. Place ground turkey in a large mixing bowl. Add sautéed vegetables, tomato sauce, egg, bread crumbs, molasses, vinegar, seasoning, basil, oregano, thyme, mustard, and black pepper. Stir with a wooden spoon or your hands until mixture is thoroughly combined.

4. Transfer meat mixture to the prepared pan and smooth top. Spread ketchup evenly over the surface. Place pan on middle rack in oven and bake 1 hour, until meatloaf is cooked through and no longer pink inside.

5. Remove from oven and serve immediately.

PER SERVING Calories: 261 | Fat: 4.9 g | Protein: 31.2 g | Sodium: 559 mg | Fiber: 2.6 g | Carbohydrates: 22.7 g | Sugar: 8.8 g

Homemade Bread Crumbs

To make your own bread crumbs, crisp several pieces of bread in the toaster or conventional oven. Tear or crumb the toasted bread into tiny pieces. For a finer crumb, pulse the bread pieces in a food processor. Wonderful bread crumb substitutes can also be made from finely chopped unsalted nuts, matzo, and salt-free potato chips.

Turkey and Quinoa Stuffed Peppers

Roasted peppers are stuffed with a delectable mixture of seasoned ground turkey, quinoa, sautéed vegetables, and beans, making each one a completely balanced meal. Red, orange, and yellow peppers are especially pretty, but green will work just fine, too. Three cups of cooked brown rice, barley, or a similar whole grain may be substituted for the cooked quinoa. Ground chicken may be used instead of turkey if desired.

PREP TIME: 10 minutes
COOK TIME: 1 hour 15 minutes

INGREDIENTS | SERVES 6

2 teaspoons olive oil, divided

3 medium red bell peppers, halved and seeded

1 cup dry quinoa, rinsed

2 cups chicken broth

1 bay leaf

1 pound lean ground turkey

1 medium onion, peeled and minced

1 medium stalk celery, trimmed and minced

3 cloves garlic, minced

3 cups chopped fresh baby spinach

1 (15-ounce) can no salt added diced tomatoes, with juice

1 (15-ounce) can black beans, drained and rinsed

1 tablespoon apple cider vinegar

1 tablespoon agave nectar

1 tablespoon ground paprika

2 teaspoons ground cumin

1 teaspoon ground coriander

1 teaspoon dried oregano

1 teaspoon all-purpose seasoning

½ teaspoon dried thyme

¼ teaspoon dried red pepper flakes

¼ cup chopped walnuts

3 tablespoons nutritional yeast

½ teaspoon freshly ground black pepper

1. Preheat oven to 375°F. Lightly oil a 9" × 13" baking pan with 1 teaspoon oil and set aside.

2. Place bell peppers cut-side up in the baking pan. Place pan on middle rack in oven and bake until tender, 30 minutes. Remove from oven and set aside.

3. Place quinoa, broth, and bay leaf in a medium saucepan and bring to a boil over high heat. Reduce heat to low, cover, and simmer until most of the liquid is absorbed and quinoa is tender, 15–20 minutes. Remove from heat, remove bay leaf, and fluff with a fork. Set aside.

4. Brown turkey in a medium skillet or sauté pan over medium heat. When turkey is almost cooked, add onion, celery, and garlic and cook, stirring, 3 minutes. Add spinach, tomatoes, and beans and cook, stirring, 3 minutes. Add vinegar, agave, paprika, cumin, coriander, oregano, seasoning, thyme, and red pepper flakes. Cook another 1–2 minutes. Remove from heat.

5. Stir quinoa into turkey mixture and mix well. Spoon filling evenly into baked peppers. Set aside.

6. Place walnuts, nutritional yeast, and 1 teaspoon oil in a food processor and pulse into a coarse crumb. Sprinkle mixture over stuffed peppers and top with black pepper.

7. Place baking pan on the middle rack in oven and bake 15 minutes, until warmed through and lightly browned on top. Remove from oven and serve immediately.

PER SERVING Calories: 362 | Fat: 7.2 g | Protein: 31.2 g | Sodium: 491 mg | Fiber: 11.4 g | Carbohydrates: 43.6 g | Sugar: 9.0 g

Lemon Thyme Turkey Meatballs

Juicy inside with a meaty outer crust, each bite of these meatballs is heightened with citrus and the heavenly scent of thyme. Serve over whole-grain noodles.

PREP TIME: 7 minutes
COOK TIME: 23 minutes

INGREDIENTS | SERVES 6

¼ cup white whole-wheat flour

1 medium onion, peeled and cut into chunks

3 cloves garlic

Grated zest of 1 medium lemon

1½ teaspoons dried thyme, divided

1 pound lean ground turkey

¾ cup bread crumbs

3 tablespoons grated Parmesan cheese

¼ teaspoon freshly ground black pepper

2 teaspoons olive oil

½ cup dry white wine

1¾ cups chicken broth

1½ tablespoons freshly squeezed lemon juice

Talking Turkey

Skinless turkey is a lean meat, containing less than 4 grams of fat per 3-ounce serving. Like chicken, it's high in vitamin B_6, protein, and minerals. Although considered a consummate holiday food, turkey consumption is on the rise in the United States as companies provide greater diversity of turkey products. Some items, such as turkey bacon and deli meats, are now being offered in healthier low-sodium versions.

1. Place flour in a shallow bowl and set aside.

2. Place onion, garlic, zest, and 1 teaspoon thyme in a food processor and pulse briefly.

3. Transfer mixture to a large bowl and mix in turkey, bread crumbs, cheese, and pepper. Pinch off 2 tablespoons at a time and shape into meatballs. Roll meatballs in flour to lightly coat. Reserve remaining flour.

4. Heat oil in a large sauté pan over medium heat. Add meatballs and cook until browned, about 5 minutes. Remove meatballs from the pan and set aside.

5. Add wine to the pan, increase heat to medium-high, and cook while scraping up any browned bits until almost evaporated, about 1 minute.

6. Add broth and bring to a boil. Reduce heat to low and return meatballs to the pan with remaining ½ teaspoon thyme. Cover and cook about 10 minutes, until meatballs are cooked through and no longer pink inside.

7. Remove meatballs again and set aside. Bring sauce to a boil over medium-high heat and cook until reduced to about 1 cup, roughly 5 minutes.

8. Add lemon juice and 1 tablespoon reserved flour into a small bowl and whisk until smooth. Add flour mixture to sauce and simmer 1–2 minutes, whisking constantly until slightly thickened. Remove from heat, add meatballs, and swirl to coat. Serve immediately.

PER SERVING Calories: 213 | Fat: 4.1 g | Protein: 22.1 g | Sodium: 554 mg | Fiber: 1.9 g | Carbohydrates: 18.0 g | Sugar: 2.2 g

CHAPTER 13

Vegetarian and Vegan

Slow Cooker Thai Red Curry

This one-pot meal is so gorgeous—like eating a rainbow!—but it's the taste that's truly fantastic. All-day simmering transforms the vegetables into a softened stew bathed in a light, spicy, citrusy coconut broth. Vary the vegetables according to what's in season or what you have on hand. Use fresh tomatoes instead of canned, cauliflower instead of broccoli, regular potatoes instead of sweet, snap peas instead of green beans, and so on. Ladle the curry over cooked brown rice, quinoa, or another whole grain.

PREP TIME: 15 minutes
COOK TIME: 5–6 hours

INGREDIENTS | SERVES 8

1 medium onion, peeled and diced

3 cloves garlic, minced

2 medium carrots, peeled and sliced

1 medium celery stalk, trimmed and sliced

2 cups chopped fresh baby spinach

8 ounces sliced fresh mushrooms

1 cup fresh green beans, cut into 1" pieces

1 medium red bell pepper, seeded and diced

1 medium head broccoli, chopped

1 medium sweet potato, peeled and diced

1 (15-ounce) can no salt added diced tomatoes, with juice

1 (15-ounce) can chickpeas, drained and rinsed

1 (15-ounce) can light coconut milk, shaken well

2 cups water

2 tablespoons Thai red curry paste

2 tablespoons low-sodium soy sauce

2 tablespoons lime juice

1 tablespoon agave nectar

2 teaspoons all-purpose seasoning

1 teaspoon ground garam masala

1 teaspoon ground coriander

½ teaspoon ground cumin

½ teaspoon freshly ground black pepper

1. Place all ingredients in a large slow cooker and stir well to combine. Cover, set to high, and cook, stirring occasionally, 5–6 hours.

2. Serve hot.

PER SERVING Calories: 156 | Fat: 3.8 g | Protein: 6.4 g | Sodium: 390 mg | Fiber: 6.6 g | Carbohydrates: 25.5 g | Sugar: 8.6 g

Hearty Vegan Lasagna

This hearty lasagna is every bit as delicious as the classic Italian version, but its ingredients make it a supremely healthy meal. Toothsome mushrooms flavor the tomato sauce, and silken tofu stands in for the ricotta cheese. For an extra-smooth filling, choose a silken variety of tofu; firm or extra-firm will work just fine, too.

PREP TIME: 15 minutes
COOK TIME: 1 hour 15 minutes

INGREDIENTS | SERVES 8

1 teaspoon olive oil

2 medium onions, peeled and chopped, divided

6 cloves garlic, minced, divided

10 ounces fresh baby bella mushrooms, chopped

1 (25-ounce) jar pasta sauce

2 teaspoons dried Italian seasoning, divided

4 tablespoons nutritional yeast, divided

1 teaspoon freshly ground black pepper, divided

½ cup vegetable broth

8 cups chopped fresh kale leaves

1 pound firm tofu, drained

1 tablespoon low-sodium soy sauce

1 teaspoon all-purpose seasoning

⅛ teaspoon dried red pepper flakes

1 (9-ounce) package oven-ready lasagna noodles

What Is Tofu?

Tofu is made from soybeans in a process not unlike the making of cheese. Bean curds are separated from liquid and pressed into blocks. Tofu is sold in two main types. The first, more perishable type must be kept cold. This tofu is submerged in liquid and comes in silken, firm, and extra-firm varieties. Silken-style tofu is sealed in shelf-stable packaging and does not need to be refrigerated. It comes in varying levels of firmness, from silken to extra-firm.

1. Preheat oven to 400°F. Get out a 9" × 13" baking pan and set aside.

2. Heat oil in a large sauté pan over medium heat. Add half the onion, half the garlic, and mushrooms. Cook, stirring, until tender, 5 minutes. Stir in pasta sauce, 1 teaspoon Italian seasoning, 1 tablespoon nutritional yeast, and ½ teaspoon black pepper. Set aside.

3. Heat broth in a large stockpot over medium heat. Add remaining onion, remaining garlic, and kale. Stir gently to combine, then cover and cook, stirring frequently, until kale has wilted completely, about 10 minutes.

4. Remove pan from heat and transfer contents to a food processor. Pulse until finely chopped. Add tofu, remaining 1 teaspoon Italian seasoning, 1 tablespoon nutritional yeast, soy sauce, all-purpose seasoning, red pepper flakes, and remaining ½ teaspoon black pepper. Pulse until smooth. Set aside.

5. To assemble the lasagna, measure roughly 1 cup sauce into the pan; spread evenly to coat. Place a layer of noodles over top. Spread ⅓ tofu filling over noodles and smooth evenly. Repeat the process with sauce, noodles, and filling until all are gone. Sprinkle remaining 2 tablespoons nutritional yeast evenly over the top.

continued on next page

6. Cover the pan with a double layer of aluminum foil; carefully pinch the sides to fully seal. Place pan on middle rack in oven and bake 1 hour, until noodles are tender.

7. Remove pan from oven, carefully remove the foil, and serve immediately.

PER SERVING Calories: 245 | Fat: 4.8 g | Protein: 13.5 g | Sodium: 515 mg | Fiber: 5.1 g | Carbohydrates: 37.8 g | Sugar: 8.0 g

Super Easy Quiche

This quiche is the perfect go-to meal for almost any occasion and always gets rave reviews. Fresh baby spinach makes prep work even easier; feel free to alter the ingredients to suit your taste, table, or pantry. The possibilities are endless.

PREP TIME: 15 minutes
COOK TIME: 1 hour

INGREDIENTS | SERVES 8

½ cup unbleached all-purpose flour

½ cup plus 2 tablespoons white whole-wheat flour, divided

5 tablespoons olive oil

2 tablespoons ice-cold water

1 medium onion, peeled and diced

2 cups sliced fresh mushrooms

4 cups chopped fresh spinach, stems removed

2 large eggs

½ cup low-fat milk

½ cup Homemade Mayonnaise (Chapter 14)

¼ teaspoon freshly ground black pepper

½ cup shredded Swiss cheese

1. Preheat oven to 350°F. Get out a 9" pie plate and set aside.

2. Place all-purpose flour and ½ cup whole-wheat flour in a medium mixing bowl and whisk well to combine. Measure oil and water into a small bowl, mix well, and pour into flour. Stir until a dough comes together, then gather dough into a ball and place between two pieces of waxed paper. Roll dough out into a large round pie crust, slightly bigger than the pie plate. Carefully transfer the pie crust to the pan; press in and patch as necessary. Set aside.

3. Heat a medium nonstick skillet over medium heat. Add onion and sauté 3 minutes. Add mushrooms and spinach and cook until onion is translucent, spinach is wilted, and mushrooms begin to release their juices, 5–7 minutes. Drain well and set aside.

4. Break eggs in a large mixing bowl and whisk well. Add milk, mayonnaise, remaining 2 tablespoons whole-wheat flour, and pepper. Blend well. Add cheese along with contents of sauté pan and stir to combine.

5. Pour filling into prepared crust. Place pan on middle rack in oven and bake 45–50 minutes until set.

6. Remove from oven, place on wire rack, and cool slightly, about 15 minutes. Serve warm or cool.

PER SERVING Calories: 297 | Fat: 22.4 g | Protein: 7.6 g | Sodium: 51 mg | Fiber: 2.2 g | Carbohydrates: 16.8 g | Sugar: 2.0 g

30-Minute Vegan Pizza

Satisfy your craving for pizza with this beautiful vegan pie. In just half an hour you'll be eating a healthy, satisfying meal that won't compromise your diet. Feeling spicy? Slice the pizza and season as desired or drizzle with hot sauce or sriracha. Swap toppings out to suit your own taste; just be sure to weigh the crust down with vegetables during the initial 15-minute baking to prevent it from ballooning up.

PREP TIME: 5 minutes
COOK TIME: 25 minutes

INGREDIENTS | SERVES 4

2 tablespoons ground flaxseed

6 tablespoons water

1½ teaspoons olive oil

1 medium onion, peeled and diced

1 medium red bell pepper, seeded and diced

1 medium green bell pepper, seeded and diced

2 cups chopped fresh kale leaves

1 cup white whole-wheat flour

1 tablespoon baking powder

1 tablespoon sugar

1 teaspoon all-purpose seasoning

1 teaspoon dried Italian seasoning

½ teaspoon garlic powder

⅔ cup unsweetened almond milk

½ cup pasta sauce

2 cloves garlic, minced

2 tablespoons chopped fresh basil

1 cup chopped fresh broccoli

½ cup sliced fresh mushrooms

1 tablespoon nutritional yeast

½ teaspoon freshly ground black pepper

Easy Greasing

The simplest way to grease and flour a pizza pan is by using olive oil cooking spray. Spray pan lightly with oil, add 1 tablespoon flour, then tap pan and tilt to disperse the flour. After the surface is evenly coated, tip pan over the sink, compost bin, or trashcan and tap lightly to remove excess flour.

1. Preheat oven to 450°F. Grease and flour a 12" pizza pan and set aside.

2. Measure flaxseed into a small bowl, add water, and stir to combine. Let rest for a few minutes to thicken.

3. Heat oil in a large sauté pan over medium heat. Add onion, bell peppers, and kale and cook, stirring, 5 minutes. Remove from heat and set aside.

4. Measure flour, baking powder, sugar, all-purpose seasoning, Italian seasoning, and garlic powder into a medium mixing bowl and whisk well to combine. Add flaxseed mixture and milk and stir just until combined. Pour batter into the prepared pizza pan and spread evenly to the edges. The dough may be a bit thick and unwieldy; just spread and smooth away holes as they arise.

5. Spoon sautéed vegetables evenly over the surface of the dough. Place pan on middle rack in oven and bake 15 minutes.

6. Remove pan from oven and spread sauce evenly over crust. Top with remaining ingredients, return to oven, and bake another 5 minutes.

7. Remove pan from oven. Cut pizza into 8 slices and serve immediately.

PER SERVING Calories: 230 | Fat: 7.6 g | Protein: 7.6 g | Sodium: 476 mg | Fiber: 7.7 g | Carbohydrates: 37.5 g | Sugar: 7.1 g

Vegetarian Gumbo

This healthy take on the classic creole dish is filled with brain-boosting vegetables and beans instead of the standard seafood. It's a deliciously modern update you're sure to love. For more tomato richness, substitute an equal amount of vegetable juice for the broth. Serve over cooked brown rice.

PREP TIME: 10 minutes
COOK TIME: 38 minutes

INGREDIENTS | SERVES 6

4 tablespoons white whole-wheat flour

3 tablespoons olive oil

1 medium onion, peeled and diced

2 medium carrots, peeled and diced

2 medium stalks celery, trimmed and diced

1 medium red bell pepper, seeded and diced

1 small green bell pepper, seeded and diced

4 cloves garlic, minced

1 (15-ounce) can no salt added diced tomatoes, with juice

1 cup vegetable broth

2½ cups fresh or frozen (thawed) okra

1 (15-ounce) can kidney beans, drained and rinsed

1 medium zucchini, diced

½ cup tomato sauce

2 bay leaves

1 teaspoon dried thyme

1 teaspoon filé powder

1 teaspoon Cajun seasoning

¼ teaspoon ground cayenne

1. Measure flour and oil into a large skillet or sauté pan and whisk well to combine. Cook, stirring constantly, over medium-low heat until brown and fragrant, 10 minutes.

2. Add the onion, carrot, celery, bell peppers, and garlic and cook, stirring, 3 minutes. Add tomatoes and vegetable broth and stir to combine. Raise heat to medium, cover, and cook 10 minutes.

3. Add remaining ingredients and stir to combine. Bring to a simmer, cover, and cook 15 minutes until vegetables are tender.

4. Remove from heat. Remove bay leaves and serve immediately.

PER SERVING Calories: 197 | Fat: 7.2 g | Protein: 7.2 g | Sodium: 615 mg | Fiber: 8.8 g | Carbohydrates: 28.3 g | Sugar: 7.3 g

What Is Filé Powder?

Filé powder, pronounced fee-lay, is a pungent seasoning made from the dried, ground leaves of the sassafras tree. Its unique flavor is added to many Cajun dishes, especially gumbo. In addition to seasoning foods, filé powder also acts as a thickening agent. It's sold at many supermarkets and online.

Savory Stuffed Acorn Squash

This tender baked squash is filled with a deliciously seasoned medley of sautéed onion, garlic, mushrooms, and spinach. It's an absolutely beautiful meal that looks and tastes impressive, but is really so easy. This makes a terrific vegetarian alternative to turkey at Thanksgiving and other holidays.

PREP TIME: 10 minutes
COOK TIME: 50 minutes

INGREDIENTS | SERVES 4

2 acorn squash, halved lengthwise, seeds and strings removed

1 tablespoon olive oil

1 medium onion, peeled and chopped

1 medium stalk celery, trimmed and chopped

3 cloves garlic, minced

1½ cups chopped fresh mushrooms

2 cups chopped fresh baby spinach

¼ cup chopped walnuts

¼ cup bread crumbs

2 tablespoons nutritional yeast

1 tablespoon low-sodium soy sauce

1 teaspoon all-purpose seasoning

1 teaspoon dried basil

¼ teaspoon dried thyme

¼ teaspoon freshly ground black pepper

1. Preheat oven to 350°F. Line a baking sheet with parchment and set aside.

2. Place squash cut-side down on the baking sheet. Place baking sheet on middle rack in oven and bake until almost tender, 30 minutes. Remove from oven and set aside.

3. Heat oil in a large sauté pan over medium heat. Add onion, celery, garlic, mushrooms, and spinach and cook, stirring, 5 minutes. Add remaining ingredients and stir well to combine. Remove pan from heat.

4. Turn squash halves over on the baking sheet and fill centers evenly with spinach mixture. Place baking sheet on middle rack in oven and bake until hot and tender, 15 minutes.

5. Remove from oven and serve immediately.

PER SERVING Calories: 195 | Fat: 8.5 g | Protein: 6.4 g | Sodium: 256 mg | Fiber: 4.5 g | Carbohydrates: 26.5 g | Sugar: 2.4 g

Ratatouille

This version of the eponymous dish mimics lasagna in arrangement and presentation and is fit to bursting with the intermingling flavors of fresh summer vegetables. If you have fresh herbs, then by all means use them; add three times the amount of any fresh herb for the dried.

PREP TIME: 15 minutes
COOK TIME: 1 hour 18 minutes

INGREDIENTS | SERVES 8

2 tablespoons olive oil

2 medium onions, peeled and diced

6 cloves garlic, minced

1 medium bell pepper, seeded and diced

1 (15-ounce) can no salt added diced tomatoes, with juice

2 (8-ounce) cans tomato sauce

2 tablespoons tomato paste

1 tablespoon agave nectar

1 tablespoon balsamic vinegar

1 teaspoon dried basil

¾ teaspoon dried marjoram

½ teaspoon dried oregano

½ teaspoon fennel seeds

½ teaspoon freshly ground black pepper

¼ teaspoon dried thyme

1 large eggplant, peeled and sliced lengthwise into strips

2 medium zucchini, sliced into thin rounds

2 medium yellow squash, sliced into thin rounds

3 tablespoons nutritional yeast

1. Preheat oven to 375°F. Get out a 9" × 13" ovensafe casserole dish and set aside.

2. Heat oil in a large skillet or sauté pan over medium heat. Add onion and garlic and sauté 3 minutes. Add bell pepper and diced tomatoes and cook, stirring, 5 minutes. Add tomato sauce, tomato paste, agave, vinegar, basil, marjoram, oregano, fennel, black pepper, and thyme; reduce heat to medium-low and simmer 10 minutes, stirring frequently. Remove from heat.

3. Assemble ratatouille in layers, similar to a lasagna. First, spoon some sauce into the bottom of the pan. Arrange eggplant over top, then cover with a thin layer of sauce. Arrange zucchini next and top with another thin layer of sauce. Then arrange squash and top with a thin layer of sauce. Repeat with any remaining vegetables; top finally with remaining sauce and nutritional yeast.

4. Cover the pan tightly with aluminum foil. Place dish on middle rack in oven and bake 1 hour, until tender and bubbling.

5. Carefully remove pan from oven and place on wire rack to cool slightly before serving. Serve hot, warm, or at room temperature.

PER SERVING Calories: 118 | Fat: 3.7 g | Protein: 4.3 g | Sodium: 331 mg | Fiber: 5.8 g | Carbohydrates: 19.4 g | Sugar: 12.1 g

Spicy Quick Noodles

This is a go-to recipe when time is tight and groceries are low. It's quick, filling, and absolutely delicious. Follow the recipe as written or vary the vegetables with whatever you have on hand; swap spinach or another dark leafy green for the broccoli, frozen green peas for the bell pepper, chopped celery for the carrot, and so on. For less spice, reduce the red pepper flakes to ¼ teaspoon. This recipe makes a very "dry" noodle; if you prefer a more liquid sauce, add additional broth.

PREP TIME: 10 minutes
COOK TIME: 10 minutes

INGREDIENTS | SERVES 6

1 (12-ounce) package whole-grain spaghetti

2 teaspoons olive oil

1 small onion, peeled and chopped

3 cloves garlic, minced

1 medium carrot, peeled and chopped

1 medium bell pepper, seeded and chopped

3 cups chopped fresh broccoli

½ cup vegetable broth

3 tablespoons apple cider vinegar

1½ tablespoons low-sodium soy sauce

1½ teaspoons ground paprika

½ teaspoon ground ginger

½ teaspoon dried red pepper flakes

⅛ teaspoon freshly ground black pepper

1. Cook spaghetti according to package directions.

2. Heat oil in a large sauté pan or skillet over medium heat. Add onion and cook, stirring, 2 minutes, until it begins to sweat. Add garlic, carrot, bell pepper, and broccoli and cook, stirring, 5 minutes, until tender. Remove pan from heat.

3. Drain pasta and add to the sauté pan. Add remaining ingredients and toss for a minute to fully coat and combine. Serve immediately.

PER SERVING Calories: 256 | Fat: 3.1 g | Protein: 9.4 g | Sodium: 239 mg | Fiber: 8.5 g | Carbohydrates: 49.7 g | Sugar: 5.1 g

Oven-Baked Spinach Burgers

These spinach- and onion-flecked burgers, filled with brain-boosting vitamin K, are perfect to eat on the MIND diet. For a vegan version, substitute 1 tablespoon ground flaxseed mixed with 3 tablespoons water for the large egg. Fresh kale may be substituted for the spinach; remove all stems, extend sautéing time by 5 minutes, and carefully drain any excess liquid. Serve with horseradish and ketchup.

PREP TIME: 10 minutes
COOK TIME: 25 minutes

INGREDIENTS | SERVES 6

2 teaspoons olive oil
1 medium onion, peeled and chopped
3 cloves garlic, minced
6 cups chopped baby spinach
1 large egg, beaten
¼ cup chopped walnuts
⅓ cup bread crumbs
3 tablespoons nutritional yeast
1 tablespoon low-sodium soy sauce
1 tablespoon white whole-wheat flour
2 teaspoons all-purpose seasoning
1 teaspoon Tabasco sauce
¼ teaspoon freshly ground black pepper

Eat Your Spinach!

Spinach is low in calories, high in fiber and protein, and an excellent source of vitamins A, B_6, C, E, and K. Just one serving of spinach a day has been shown to slow cognitive decline. Spinach is easy to grow in home gardens year-round, and can be frozen for later use. It's delicious in both savory dishes as well as sweet drinks, like fruit smoothies, making it a great addition to almost any meal. Other ways to incorporate more spinach into your diet: instead of lettuce in your sandwiches substitute fresh baby spinach, or chop and stir into soups, stews, curries, or pilafs for an added burst of nutrients.

1. Preheat oven to 375°F. Line a baking sheet with parchment and set aside.

2. Heat oil in a large sauté pan over medium heat. Add onion and cook, stirring, 2 minutes, until it begins to sweat. Add garlic and spinach and cook, stirring, 3 minutes until wilted. Remove pan from heat and transfer contents to a medium mixing bowl.

3. Add remaining ingredients to the bowl and stir well to combine. Scoop mixture out by roughly ¼ cup and form into patties. Mixture will be sticky; wash hands as necessary.

4. Place patties on the baking sheet. Place sheet on middle rack in oven and bake 10 minutes. Gently flip patties over and bake another 10 minutes, until firm and lightly golden.

5. Remove from oven and serve immediately.

PER SERVING Calories: 111 | Fat: 5.7 g | Protein: 5.3 g | Sodium: 218 mg | Fiber: 2.2 g | Carbohydrates: 10.2 g | Sugar: 1.4 g

Peanut Butter Noodles

This noodle dish is quick, easy, inexpensive, and perfect for busy weeknight dinners. It comes together as quickly as you can cook the pasta, and can be bulked up with whatever sautéed vegetables or dark leafy greens you have on hand. If you don't have tahini, add an extra tablespoon of peanut butter.

PREP TIME: 5 minutes
COOK TIME: 10 minutes

INGREDIENTS | SERVES 6

1 (12-ounce) package whole-grain spaghetti

1 cup vegetable broth

1 tablespoon apple cider vinegar

1½ tablespoons low-sodium soy sauce

3 tablespoons peanut butter

1 tablespoon tahini

2 cloves garlic, minced

2 teaspoons agave nectar

1½ teaspoons Tabasco sauce

½ cup chopped fresh cilantro

⅛ teaspoon freshly ground black pepper

1. Cook spaghetti according to package directions.

2. Measure broth, vinegar, soy sauce, peanut butter, tahini, garlic, agave, and Tabasco into a small saucepan. Place over low heat and whisk until smooth. Remove from heat.

3. Drain pasta and return to pot. Pour sauce over pasta; use a spatula to scrape everything out of the saucepan. Add cilantro and pepper to pot and toss for a minute to coat pasta completely. Serve immediately.

PER SERVING Calories: 277 | Fat: 6.7 g | Protein: 9.7 g | Sodium: 339 mg | Fiber: 6.9 g | Carbohydrates: 46.7 g | Sugar: 4.9 g

Slow Cooker Cilantro, Potato, and Pea Curry

This dish is made up of tender potatoes and peas simmered in a delicious coconut-scented tomato broth. Serve this over cooked brown rice for an extra-hearty, healthy meal. The recipe calls for vegetable juice; substitute vegetable broth instead if desired.

PREP TIME: 15 minutes
COOK TIME: 6 hours

INGREDIENTS | SERVES 8

1 large onion, peeled and diced

6 cloves garlic, minced

2 cups vegetable juice

1 (15-ounce) can light coconut milk

6 tablespoons tomato paste

8 medium potatoes, peeled and cut into 1" cubes

3 cups fresh or frozen green peas

2 tablespoons low-sodium soy sauce

2 tablespoons natural (unflavored) rice wine vinegar

2 tablespoons curry powder

1 tablespoon agave nectar

1 teaspoon ground ginger

¼ teaspoon freshly ground black pepper

⅓ cup chopped fresh cilantro

1. Place all ingredients except cilantro in a slow cooker. Stir well to combine, cover, and cook on high 6 hours.

2. Stir in cilantro and serve immediately.

PER SERVING Calories: 263 | Fat: 3.5 g | Protein: 8.7 g | Sodium: 534 mg | Fiber: 7.8 g | Carbohydrates: 50.5 g | Sugar: 9.8 g

Tell Me More about Turmeric

Turmeric is a spice made from the ground root of the turmeric plant. Its bright yellow color and distinct flavor are used in many types of food, from Indian curries and curry powder to classic American prepared mustard. Turmeric has a slightly bitter taste that works well in combination with other seasonings. It's high in manganese and iron, and may help reduce the risk of certain types of cancer.

Spicy Pan-Roasted Chickpeas with Tahini Sauce

Addictively delicious, these highly seasoned chickpeas are served atop fresh greens and drizzled with a tangy tahini dressing. Chopped kale, baby spinach, or arugula may be substituted for (or added to) the salad greens if desired. For another variation, serve the chickpeas, dressing, and greens in warmed soft tortillas or crunchy taco shells.

PREP TIME: 5 minutes
COOK TIME: 6 minutes

INGREDIENTS | SERVES 6

4 tablespoons tahini

3 tablespoons water

3½ tablespoons lemon juice, divided

2 tablespoons olive oil, divided

1 tablespoon natural (unflavored) rice wine vinegar

2 teaspoons low-sodium soy sauce, divided

2 cloves garlic, minced

2 (15-ounce) cans chickpeas, drained and rinsed

1 teaspoon agave nectar

2 teaspoons ground paprika

2 teaspoons ground cumin

1 teaspoon garlic powder

¼ teaspoon ground cayenne

⅛ teaspoon freshly ground black pepper

6 cups fresh spring mix

1. To make the dressing, measure tahini into a small mixing bowl. Add water, 1½ tablespoons lemon juice, 1 tablespoon oil, vinegar, 1 teaspoon soy sauce, and garlic. Whisk well to combine. Sauce may be made ahead and refrigerated until serving.

2. Heat remaining 1 tablespoon oil in a large sauté pan over medium-high heat. Add chickpeas and cook, stirring, 5 minutes, until they begin to sizzle. Add remaining 2 tablespoons lemon juice, remaining 1 teaspoon soy sauce, agave nectar, paprika, cumin, garlic powder, cayenne and pepper and cook, stirring, 1 minute, until coated and tender.

3. Remove pan from heat. Spoon chickpeas over greens and drizzle with tahini sauce. Serve immediately.

PER SERVING Calories: 230 | Fat: 11.2 g | Protein: 8.7 g | Sodium: 279 mg | Fiber: 7.3 g | Carbohydrates: 26.1 g | Sugar: 4.6 g

Make-Your-Own Black Bean Burgers

Making this dish is almost as easy as opening a box of frozen veggie burgers, but so much better for you! The combination of nuts, beans, and vital wheat gluten gives these burgers a heft and chew that's irresistible. Substitute any type of unsalted nuts or sunflower seeds for the walnuts if desired. Instead of oven-baking, these burgers may also be pan-fried on the stovetop; heat 1 cup olive oil in a skillet over medium and brown burgers on both sides until brown and crispy, 2–4 minutes per side.

PREP TIME: 5 minutes
COOK TIME: 30 minutes

INGREDIENTS | SERVES 4

½ cup walnuts
1 (15-ounce) can black beans, drained and rinsed
1 small onion, peeled and quartered
2 tablespoons low-sodium soy sauce
2 teaspoons all-purpose seasoning
1 teaspoon ground paprika
¼ teaspoon freshly ground black pepper
⅓ cup vital wheat gluten

What Is Vital Wheat Gluten?

Gluten is the natural protein found in wheat. It's what gives bread its beloved dense chew. Vital wheat gluten is the powdered form of this gluten—basically wheat protein in a box—which can be added to breads and other recipes to make them chewier. It's sold in the baking aisle of most supermarkets, alongside the flour and sugar, and in many natural food stores. Vital wheat gluten looks like flour, and feels like flour, but once it's incorporated with liquids, it becomes so much more. Buy in bulk and store in the freezer for longevity.

1. Place nuts in a food processor and pulse until finely chopped.

2. Add beans, onion, soy sauce, seasoning, paprika, and pepper and pulse until smooth.

3. Add wheat gluten and process until mixture comes together to form a firm dough. The mixture should gather up and spin as a cohesive ball. Test the firmness with a fingertip. If the dough is still sticky or isn't coming together well, add a little additional wheat gluten 1–2 tablespoons at a time until it firms up and is easy to handle.

4. Remove firm dough from the food processor and roll into a tight ball. Place on clean surface and cut in half, then half again, to form 4 equal wedges. Roll each fourth into a ball, then press to form a patty.

5. Preheat oven to 350°F. Line a baking sheet with parchment and arrange patties several inches apart. Place tray on middle rack and bake 12–15 minutes, then remove tray, flip patties, and return to bake another 12–15 minutes. To achieve a crisper crust, spray or brush the burgers lightly with olive oil before baking.

6. Serve immediately.

PER SERVING Calories: 237 | Fat: 9.4 g | Protein: 18.2 g | Sodium: 393 mg | Fiber: 9.1 g | Carbohydrates: 20.8 g | Sugar: 2.2 g

Amazing Vegetable Casserole with Tofu Topping

This recipe makes great use of some of the healthiest and least expensive vegetables: carrots, onions, cabbage, and kale. Best of all, they're abundantly available year-round. Sandwiched under a crust of crumbled tofu, bread crumbs, and chopped nuts, this dish is an incredible casserole with tons of taste and texture.

PREP TIME: 10 minutes
COOK TIME: 35 minutes

INGREDIENTS | SERVES 8

3 tablespoons olive oil, divided
2 medium onions, peeled and thinly sliced
½ medium head green cabbage, sliced
1 pound chopped fresh kale leaves
3 medium carrots, peeled and sliced into thin sticks
½ cup vegetable broth
2 tablespoons low-sodium soy sauce
1½ cups bread crumbs
8 ounces extra-firm tofu, drained
¼ cup chopped walnuts
3 cloves garlic
2 tablespoons nutritional yeast
2 teaspoons dried basil
1½ teaspoons dried oregano
1 teaspoon ground paprika
¼ teaspoon freshly ground black pepper

Walnut Facts

Walnuts have a wonderfully nutty flavor that complements everything from baked goods to salads and entrées. They're rich in monounsaturated fats and omega-3 fatty acids, manganese, and copper, and have been shown to prevent cardiovascular disease, lower cholesterol, and protect against certain types of cancer. Most importantly on the MIND diet, walnuts have been proven to aid in memory retention and strengthen motor development. Walnuts are even shaped just like miniature brains!

1. Preheat oven to 350°F. Get out a 9" × 13" ovensafe baking dish and set aside.

2. Heat 1 tablespoon oil in a large skillet or sauté pan over medium heat. Add onions and cook, stirring, until softened, 3 minutes. Add cabbage, kale, carrots, broth, and soy sauce. Skillet will be very full; volume will reduce as vegetables cook. Cover the pan and cook, stirring occasionally, until vegetables are just tender, 12 minutes. Transfer contents to the baking dish and set aside.

3. To make the topping, measure remaining 2 tablespoons oil bread crumbs, tofu, walnuts, garlic, nutritional yeast, basil, oregano, paprika, and pepper into a food processor and pulse to combine. Alternatively, mash ingredients together in a large bowl with a potato masher.

4. Sprinkle tofu mixture over vegetables in baking dish. Place dish on middle rack in oven and bake uncovered until topping is golden brown and vegetables are heated through, 15–20 minutes.

5. Remove from oven and serve immediately.

PER SERVING Calories: 244 | Fat: 9.9 g | Protein: 10.6 g | Sodium: 540 mg | Fiber: 6.5 g | Carbohydrates: 30.4 g | Sugar: 5.2 g

Lemon Pesto Rice with Portobello Mushrooms

This recipe gives you a hearty vegan one-dish meal perfect for weeknights and potluck parties. The bright bite of lemon pesto is fabulous on its own, but partnered with sautéed onion, meaty mushrooms, and brown rice, it's downright addictive. This recipe works equally well with cooked whole-grain pasta, quinoa, and other grains. For the pesto, use your favorite type of unsalted nuts: walnuts, pecans, almonds, or cashews.

PREP TIME: 10 minutes
COOK TIME: 10 minutes

INGREDIENTS | SERVES 6

2½ tablespoons olive oil, divided

1 large onion, peeled and chopped

16 ounces baby bella mushrooms, chopped

6 cups cooked brown rice

Juice of 2 medium lemons

6 cloves garlic

1½ teaspoons agave nectar

½ teaspoon mustard

⅓ cup chopped walnuts

⅓ cup fresh basil leaves, packed

2 tablespoons nutritional yeast

1 teaspoon all-purpose seasoning

¼ teaspoon freshly ground black pepper

1. Heat 1 tablespoon oil in a large stockpot over medium heat. Add onion and mushrooms and cook, stirring, 10 minutes, until tender. Remove from heat, stir in cooked rice, cover, and set aside.

2. Measure remaining 1½ tablespoons oil, lemon juice, garlic, agave, mustard, nuts, basil, nutritional yeast, seasoning, and pepper into a food processor and pulse until smooth.

3. Stir pesto into rice mixture until well combined. Serve immediately.

PER SERVING Calories: 352 | Fat: 11.1 g | Protein: 8.6 g | Sodium: 14 mg | Fiber: 5.3 g | Carbohydrates: 55.6 g | Sugar: 4.0 g

For Fun and Freshness, Grow Your Own!

Fresh herbs are easy and inexpensive to grow in almost any living situation. A sunny windowsill or patio planter can produce enough herbs to flavor a wide array of recipes any time of year. A few bargain pots, some soil, and seeds are all you need to get started. Enjoy your favorite herbs at their freshest by growing your own!

Speedy Samosa Pasta

In this dish, whole-grain spaghetti is tossed with diced potato and green peas and coated in a flavorful curry sauce. It's like a healthy bowl of samosas in less than 30 minutes! Your mind will thank you!

PREP TIME: 10 minutes
COOK TIME: 15 minutes

INGREDIENTS | SERVES 6

1 (12-ounce) package whole-grain spaghetti

2 medium potatoes, scrubbed and pierced with a fork

1 tablespoon olive oil

1 medium onion, peeled and chopped

3 cloves garlic, minced

1 cup frozen green peas, thawed

1 cup vegetable broth

2 tablespoons apple cider vinegar

1½ tablespoons low-sodium soy sauce

1 teaspoon agave nectar

3 tablespoons nutritional yeast

2 teaspoons curry powder

1 teaspoon all-purpose seasoning

1 teaspoon ground paprika

¼ teaspoon dried red pepper flakes

⅛ teaspoon freshly ground black pepper

¼ cup chopped fresh cilantro

1. Cook pasta according to package directions.

2. Place potatoes in the microwave and cook 4 minutes on high, turn over, and cook another 4 minutes. Insert a paring knife into the potatoes to check for doneness. If knife slides in smoothly, potato is done; if not, microwave in 30-second increments until done. Remove potatoes from microwave, let rest briefly to cool, then dice.

3. Heat oil in a large skillet or sauté pan over medium heat. Add onion and sauté 2 minutes, until it begins to sweat. Add garlic and green peas and cook, stirring, 1 minute. Add remaining ingredients except pasta and cilantro and cook, stirring, until sauce has thickened slightly, 3–4 minutes.

4. Drain pasta and return to pot. Add potato. Pour sauce over top, add cilantro, and toss well to combine. Serve immediately.

PER SERVING Calories: 315 | Fat: 4.0 g | Protein: 11.4 g | Sodium: 387 mg | Fiber: 9.6 g | Carbohydrates: 60.5 g | Sugar: 5.6 g

Meatless Meatloaf

This meatless meatloaf is moist, melt-in-your-mouth comfort food—pure deliciousness with absolutely no guilt! If you're not happy with store-bought condiments, recipes for homemade ketchup, barbecue sauce, and mustard are in Chapter 14.

PREP TIME: 20 minutes
COOK TIME: 53 minutes

INGREDIENTS | SERVES 6

3 teaspoons olive oil, divided

3 medium potatoes, scrubbed and cubed

1 (15-ounce) can kidney beans, drained and rinsed

1 medium bell pepper, seeded and chopped

1 medium onion, peeled and chopped

3 cloves garlic, minced

2 teaspoons ground cumin

1 teaspoon chili seasoning

1½ cups quick oats

½ cup barbecue sauce, divided

¼ cup ketchup

2½ teaspoons mustard

½ teaspoon freshly ground black pepper

¼ cup chopped fresh cilantro

2 tablespoons nutritional yeast

1. Preheat oven to 375°F. Lightly oil an 8" square pan with 1 teaspoon oil and set aside.

2. Place potatoes in a large saucepan. Add enough water to cover, bring to a boil over high heat, then reduce heat slightly and cook until tender, roughly 15 minutes. Drain and mash potatoes. Set aside.

3. Mash beans using the tines of a fork and set aside.

4. Heat 2 teaspoons oil in a skillet over medium heat. Add bell pepper, onion, garlic, cumin, and chili seasoning and cook, stirring, 3 minutes, until they begin to sweat. Remove from heat. Stir in potatoes, beans, oats, ¼ cup barbecue sauce, ketchup, mustard, black pepper, and cilantro.

5. Spoon mixture into prepared pan and smooth top to even. Spread remaining barbecue sauce over top and sprinkle with nutritional yeast.

6. Place pan on middle rack in oven and bake 35 minutes, until hot and steaming. Remove from oven, let rest 10 minutes, slice, and serve warm.

PER SERVING Calories: 292 | Fat: 4.0 g | Protein: 9.9 g | Sodium: 481 mg | Fiber: 8.0 g | Carbohydrates: 55.2 g | Sugar: 12.1 g

CHAPTER 14

Sauces and Dressings

Special 6-in-1 Roasting Sauce

This intensely flavorful, spicy-sweet sauce transforms roasted vegetables into irresistible treats. Whisk together, drizzle over your choice of vegetables, toss, and bake. It's delicious on everything from Brussels sprouts and green beans to sweet potatoes and winter squash. It also makes a great brush-on grilling sauce for lean meats and tofu.

PREP TIME: 2 minutes
COOK TIME: N/A

INGREDIENTS | YIELDS ⅓ CUP

1 tablespoon agave nectar
1 tablespoon apple cider vinegar
1 tablespoon lime juice
1 tablespoon low-sodium soy sauce
1 tablespoon olive oil
1 tablespoon sriracha

1. Place all ingredients in a small bowl and whisk well to combine.

2. Use immediately or store in an airtight container, refrigerate, and use within 2 days.

PER 1-TABLESPOON SERVING Calories: 52 | Fat: 3.3 g | Protein: 0.3 g | Sodium: 187 mg | Fiber: 0.3 g | Carbohydrates: 5.3 g | Sugar: 4.6 g

Spinach-Walnut Pesto

This scrumptious pesto can be used in a myriad of ways. Stir it into cooked pasta, brown rice, quinoa, or another whole grain. Use it as a spread for sandwiches, crackers, or pizza. Or partner it with raw vegetables and hummus for a party tray. For variety, substitute fresh arugula for the baby spinach.

PREP TIME: 3 minutes

COOK TIME: N/A

INGREDIENTS | YIELDS 1 CUP

2 cups packed fresh basil leaves

1 cup packed fresh baby spinach

¼ cup walnuts

3 cloves garlic

3 tablespoons nutritional yeast

3 tablespoons olive oil

1 tablespoon lemon juice

1 tablespoon low-sodium soy sauce

¼ teaspoon freshly ground black pepper

1. Place all ingredients in a food processor and pulse until smooth.

2. Use immediately or store in an airtight container, refrigerate, and use within 2 days.

PER 1-TABLESPOON SERVING Calories: 48 | Fat: 4.5 g | Protein: 1.1 g | Sodium: 42 mg | Fiber: 0.5 g | Carbohydrates: 1.2 g | Sugar: 0.1 g

Asian Peanut Sauce

This Asian Peanut Sauce is a creamy, tangy, absolutely delicious dressing for salads and bowl meals. This can be tossed with raw or roasted vegetables, whole-grain pasta, quinoa, and more, or used as a dip for grilled meat or tofu. It's so good, you may just want to eat it by the spoon.

PREP TIME: 5 minutes
COOK TIME: N/A

INGREDIENTS | YIELDS ½ CUP

3 tablespoons peanut butter

2 tablespoons lime juice

1 tablespoon tahini

1 tablespoon apple cider vinegar

2 teaspoons low-sodium soy sauce

2 cloves garlic, minced

½ teaspoons agave nectar

¼ teaspoon ground ginger

1. Place all ingredients in a small bowl and whisk well to combine.

2. Use immediately or store in an airtight container, refrigerate, and use within 2 days.

PER 1-TABLESPOON SERVING Calories: 58 | Fat: 4.4 g | Protein: 2.1 g | Sodium: 77 mg | Fiber: 0.6 g | Carbohydrates: 3.2 g | Sugar: 1.2 g

What Is Vinegar?

Vinegar is produced when an alcoholic liquid is allowed to ferment and the ethanol within it oxidizes. The remaining liquid becomes highly acidic and is what we refer to as vinegar. Balsamic vinegar is made from the leftover pressings (called must) of white grapes that are first boiled down to form a syrup and then allowed to age. Apple cider vinegar is made from a similar process using apple must. Rice wine vinegar is made by fermenting the sugars in rice into an alcohol and then allowing it to age into acid.

Lemon-Dill Sauce

A delicious dressing for vegetables, green salads, and seafood, this bright and creamy sauce has a lively citrus kick. Kelp granules are sold with the herbs and spices in many supermarkets and natural food stores. When available, use 1 teaspoon chopped fresh dill instead of the dried.

PREP TIME: 2 minutes
COOK TIME: N/A

INGREDIENTS | YIELDS ⅓ CUP

2 tablespoons lemon juice

2 tablespoons olive oil

1 tablespoon nutritional yeast

½ teaspoon all-purpose seasoning

¼ teaspoon dried dill

¼ teaspoon dried herbes de Provence

¼ teaspoon kelp granules

1. Place all ingredients in a small bowl and whisk well to combine.

2. Use immediately or store in an airtight container, refrigerate, and use within 2 days.

PER 1-TABLESPOON SERVING Calories: 65 | Fat: 6.6 g | Protein: 0.6 g | Sodium: 8 mg | Fiber: 0.3 g | Carbohydrates: 1.0 g | Sugar: 0.2 g

Orange Cranberry Sauce

Cranberries, orange juice, and fresh clementine come together in this sweet and tart sauce great for holiday dining and so much more. This thick relish is superb year-round as a sandwich topping, addition to breakfast, or garnish for roasted meat.

PREP TIME: 5 minutes
COOK TIME: 10 minutes

INGREDIENTS | YIELDS 2 CUPS

1 cup orange juice

1 cup sugar

3 cups fresh whole cranberries, washed and drained

1 clementine, peeled, segmented, and chopped

Cranberry Facts

Cranberries contain antioxidants and high levels of vitamin C, and have been reported to inhibit cancer. But what they're best known for is their ability to protect against urinary tract infections. A substance within the cranberry is thought to prevent bacteria from adhering to the bladder wall, thus preventing attack. Fresh cranberries are sold during the fall and winter holidays; buy an extra bag or two and store in the freezer. When frozen, cranberries will keep well for many months. Thaw before using.

1. Place juice and sugar in a small saucepan or small stockpot and stir to combine. Bring to a boil over high heat.

2. Add cranberries and clementine, reduce heat to medium, and simmer 10 minutes, until tender. Sauce will thicken significantly as it cools, so if it appears thin, don't be concerned.

3. Remove from heat, cover, and cool. Serve at room temperature.

PER 1-TABLESPOON SERVING Calories: 39 | Fat: 0.0 g | Protein: 0.1 g | Sodium: 0 mg | Fiber: 0.6 g | Carbohydrates: 10.1 g | Sugar: 8.9 g

Avocado Whip

This creamy, dreamy avocado dressing is like a spicy, lime-spiked vegan mayonnaise. It's light, whipped, and fantastically flavorful! Turn any salad into a Southwestern sensation by spooning and tossing with this delicious green dressing. Dollop over nachos or tacos, spread in burritos, or serve with salsa as a dip for tortilla chips. It makes a fabulous sandwich spread and is even great alone on toast.

PREP TIME: 5 minutes
COOK TIME: N/A

INGREDIENTS | YIELDS ⅔ CUP

½ ripe medium avocado, pitted and flesh removed

3 cloves garlic, minced

2 tablespoons tahini

2 tablespoons lime juice

1 tablespoon apple cider vinegar

1 tablespoon water

1½ teaspoons agave nectar

½ teaspoon ground coriander

⅛ teaspoon ground cayenne

1. Place all ingredients in a food processor and pulse until smooth.

2. Serve immediately or store in an airtight container, refrigerate, and use within 2 days.

PER 1-TABLESPOON SERVING Calories: 38 | Fat: 2.8 g | Protein: 0.8 g | Sodium: 4 mg | Fiber: 1.0 g | Carbohydrates: 3.0 g | Sugar: 1.0 g

Grapefruit Vinaigrette

This Grapefruit Vinaigrette is a light and refreshing dressing with a tangy-sweet taste. Half of a medium-sized grapefruit should yield 4 tablespoons of juice; use bottled juice if you don't have fresh fruit. Ruby red grapefruit makes a pink dressing as delicious as it is pretty. Drizzle over a mixture of greens, chickpeas, fruit, and sunflower seeds.

PREP TIME: 3 minutes
COOK TIME: N/A

INGREDIENTS | YIELDS ½ CUP

4 tablespoons grapefruit juice

2 tablespoons olive oil

1 tablespoon agave nectar

2 teaspoons red wine vinegar

2 cloves garlic, minced

½ teaspoon dried marjoram

⅛ teaspoon dried thyme

⅛ teaspoon ground rosemary

⅛ teaspoon freshly ground black pepper

1. Place all ingredients in a small bowl and whisk well to combine.

2. Use immediately or store in an airtight container, refrigerate, and use within 2 days.

PER 1-TABLESPOON SERVING Calories: 47 | Fat: 3.8 g | Protein: 0.1 g | Sodium: 0 mg | Fiber: 0.2 g | Carbohydrates: 3.5 g | Sugar: 2.2 g

Grapefruit Facts

Grapefruit is a subtropical citrus fruit that originated in Barbados as a cross between a sweet orange and a pomelo, both originally from Asia. Once called "the forbidden fruit," grapefruit is now widely available and is classified by the color of its inner flesh, either white, pink, or red. Grapefruit comes in a range of varieties, some sweet, some much more tartly sour. All varieties contain high levels of vitamin C and antioxidants, as well as lower levels of vitamins A and B_6, and copper. Red and pink grapefruit also contain lycopene, a phytonutrient believed to combat cancer.

Balsamic Vinaigrette

The combination of balsamic and red wine vinegars lightens the intensity of this classic dressing. The recipes yields ¼ cup, enough for 4 servings; double or triple the ingredients for a larger party-sized salad.

PREP TIME: 3 minutes
COOK TIME: N/A

INGREDIENTS | YIELDS ¼ CUP

2 tablespoons olive oil
1 tablespoon balsamic vinegar
1 tablespoon red wine vinegar
1 clove garlic, minced
1 teaspoon agave nectar
1 teaspoon ground mustard
¼ teaspoon dried Italian seasoning
⅛ teaspoon freshly ground black pepper

1. Place all ingredients in a small bowl and whisk well to combine.

2. Use immediately or store in an airtight container, refrigerate, and use within 2 days.

PER 1-TABLESPOON SERVING Calories: 96 | Fat: 9.0 g | Protein: 0.3 g | Sodium: 1 mg | Fiber: 0.2 g | Carbohydrates: 3.3 g | Sugar: 2.5 g

Tomato Garlic Dressing

If you're someone who puts ketchup on everything, here's the dressing of your dreams! With its vibrant color and tangy taste, it's great drizzled over salad or served with grilled vegetables, meats, and sandwiches. If you don't have white pepper, substitute ¼ teaspoon freshly ground black pepper instead.

PREP TIME: 2 minutes
COOK TIME: N/A

INGREDIENTS | YIELDS ⅓ CUP

2 tablespoons red wine vinegar

2 tablespoons lemon juice

1 tablespoon tomato paste

1½ teaspoons olive oil

2 cloves garlic

1 teaspoon agave nectar

⅛ teaspoon ground white pepper

1. Place all ingredients in a food processor and pulse until smooth.

2. Serve immediately or store in an airtight container, refrigerate, and use within 2 days.

PER 1-TABLESPOON SERVING Calories: 27 | Fat: 1.7 g | Protein: 0.3 g | Sodium: 32 mg | Fiber: 0.3 g | Carbohydrates: 3.2 g | Sugar: 1.9 g

Homemade Dressing

Store-bought salad dressings offer convenience, but at what cost? Most are filled with fat, excess sodium, and unrecognizable ingredients. Instead of buying commercial dressings, spend money on new and interesting vinegars, oils, and fruit juices. Add garlic, scallions, or shallot, fresh or dried herbs, ground or prepared mustard, some spice, and you've got a world of flavor in mere minutes.

Mango Salsa

Ripe mangoes, garlic, lime, and cilantro flavor one of the most mouthwateringly tasty salsas ever. When mangoes are out of season, substitute an equal amount of fresh or canned pineapple chunks. Be creative with the recipe and try it out with other fruits, like fresh strawberries, ripe peaches, and garden-ripe tomatoes.

PREP TIME: 7 minutes
COOK TIME: N/A

INGREDIENTS | YIELDS 2 CUPS

1 ripe mango, peeled, cored, and diced

1 medium red bell pepper, seeded and chopped

2 cloves garlic, minced

1 jalapeño pepper, seeded and minced

Juice of 1 medium lime

¼ cup chopped fresh cilantro

1 tablespoon apple cider vinegar

1 teaspoon agave nectar

1 teaspoon ground cumin

1. Place all ingredients in a medium mixing bowl and stir well to combine.

2. Serve immediately or store in an airtight container, refrigerate, and use within 2 days.

PER 1-TABLESPOON SERVING Calories: 10 | Fat: 0.1 g | Protein: 0.2 g | Sodium: 0 mg | Fiber: 0.3 g | Carbohydrates: 2.5 g | Sugar: 2.1 g

Selecting a Ripe Mango

When selecting fresh mangoes, follow your nose. Sniff the stem end of the mango for clues to ripeness. Still in doubt? Let your fingers be your guide. Ripe mangoes will yield to gentle pressure, less ripe will give only a little, and unripe will remain hard. Select fruit with smooth, unblemished skin. And don't be fooled by the color of the peel; it has nothing to do with ripeness.

Simply Delicious Pasta Sauce

This chunky vegetable-packed tomato sauce is so flavorful! Delicious, healthy, and so easy to make, you may never buy the jarred stuff again. It freezes well too, so feel free to double the recipe and store in an airtight container in the freezer for up to 2 months; thaw before serving.

PREP TIME: 10 minutes
COOK TIME: 30 minutes

INGREDIENTS | YIELDS 8 CUPS

2 tablespoons olive oil

1 medium onion, peeled and chopped

1 medium bell pepper, seeded and chopped

2 medium carrots, peeled and chopped

2 medium stalks celery, trimmed and chopped

6 cloves garlic, minced

8 ounces fresh mushrooms, chopped

2 cups chopped baby spinach, packed

1 (15-ounce) can no salt added diced tomatoes

3 (8-ounce) cans tomato sauce

4 tablespoons tomato paste

¼ cup red wine

2 tablespoons nutritional yeast

1½ tablespoons agave nectar

2 teaspoons all-purpose seasoning

2 teaspoons dried basil

1 teaspoon dried oregano

1 teaspoon fennel seeds

½ teaspoon dried marjoram

½ teaspoon dried thyme

¼ freshly ground black pepper

⅛ teaspoon dried red pepper flakes

1. Heat oil in a large sauté pan over medium heat. Add onion and cook, stirring, 2 minutes. Add bell pepper, carrots, celery, garlic, mushrooms, and spinach and cook, stirring, 5 minutes, until spinach has wilted and vegetables are starting to brown.

2. Add remaining ingredients and stir well to combine. Cook until the mixture begins to bubble, then reduce heat to low, cover, and simmer 23 minutes, stirring occasionally, until thick and chunky.

3. Remove from heat. Serve immediately or store in an airtight container, refrigerate, and use within 3 days.

PER 1-CUP SERVING Calories: 144 | Fat: 4.8 g | Protein: 4.8 g | Sodium: 608 mg | Fiber: 6.4 g | Carbohydrates: 24.0 g | Sugar: 12.8 g

Homemade Mayonnaise

This light and creamy mayonnaise uses a liquid egg substitute, eliminating both cholesterol and the risk of salmonella. Make this recipe ahead when you have time; Homemade Mayonnaise keeps well for a week if stored in a clean, airtight jar in the refrigerator. Adjust seasonings to suit your own taste.

PREP TIME: 5 minutes
COOK TIME: N/A

INGREDIENTS | YIELDS 1 CUP

¼ cup liquid egg substitute

2½ tablespoons distilled white vinegar

½ teaspoon ground white pepper

⅛ teaspoon garlic powder

⅛ teaspoon ground mustard

¹⁄₁₆ teaspoon ground cayenne

⅔ cup olive oil

1. Place egg substitute, vinegar, pepper, garlic powder, mustard, and cayenne in a food processor and pulse until smooth. Scrape down the sides.

2. With food processor running, add oil in a slow and steady stream until mixture thickens.

3. Store mayonnaise in a clean lidded jar, refrigerate, and use within a week.

PER 1-TABLESPOON SERVING Calories: 100 | Fat: 10.8 | Protein: 0.5 g | Sodium: 9 mg | Fiber: 0.0 g | Carbohydrates: 0.2 g | Sugar: 0.1 g

Liquid Egg Substitute

Sold in cartons alongside eggs, liquid egg substitutes such as Egg Beaters are a great way of enjoying the flavor of whole eggs without the fat and cholesterol. In most recipes, you can use ¼ cup of liquid egg substitute for each egg without a discernible difference in taste or texture. Liquid egg substitutes can be frozen as well, making them both healthy and convenient.

Homemade Honey Mustard

This delicious mustard takes only 5 minutes to prepare and yields a sweet and zingy mustard as good as any gourmet brand.

PREP TIME: 2 minutes
COOK TIME: 5 minutes

INGREDIENTS | YIELDS ¾ CUP

½ cup ground mustard
½ cup distilled white vinegar
¼ cup honey
1 tablespoon olive oil
¼ teaspoon ground allspice
¼ teaspoon garlic powder
¼ teaspoon freshly ground black pepper

Chef's Note

Homemade mustard will thicken significantly when refrigerated, so don't be concerned if it appears somewhat loose right after the cooking time has ended. Homemade mustard will keep for weeks in the refrigerator. Store in a clean lidded jar, labeled with the date if possible.

1. Combine all ingredients in a small saucepan. Place over medium-high heat and stir constantly until boiling.

2. Reduce heat to medium-low and simmer until mustard begins to thicken, roughly 5 minutes.

3. Pour into a clean lidded jar, refrigerate, and use within a month. Mustard will thicken significantly in the refrigerator, so if it appears thin initially don't be concerned.

PER 1-TABLESPOON SERVING Calories: 65 | Fat: 3.1 g | Protein: 1.4 g | Sodium: 1 mg | Fiber: 0.6 g | Carbohydrates: 8.4 g | Sugar: 7.2 g

Homemade Ketchup

There's no need to purchase commercial ketchup when it's this easy to make at home. This ketchup contains no artificial additives, preservatives, or sweeteners, and it's delicious! Season to taste as desired.

PREP TIME: 2 minutes
COOK TIME: 10 minutes

INGREDIENTS | YIELDS 3 CUPS

3 (8-ounce) cans tomato sauce

5 tablespoons tomato paste

3 tablespoons distilled white vinegar

5 teaspoons sugar

¼ teaspoon garlic powder

¼ teaspoon onion powder

⅛ teaspoon ground mustard

⅛ teaspoon ground cinnamon

⅛ teaspoon ground cumin

1. Measure all ingredients into a large saucepan and stir until completely smooth.

2. Place pan over medium heat. As soon as the mixture begins to bubble, reduce heat to low and simmer 10 minutes.

3. Remove from heat and pour ketchup into a clean lidded jar, refrigerate, and use within a month.

PER 1-TABLESPOON SERVING Calories: 8 | Fat: 0.0 g | Protein: 0.3 g | Sodium: 96 mg | Fiber: 0.4 g | Carbohydrates: 1.9 g | Sugar: 1.4 g

Spicy, Sweet, and Tangy Barbecue Sauce

Fat-free and absolutely amazing, this authentic-tasting barbecue sauce is perfect for all of your grilling, basting, and dipping needs. If stored in the refrigerator, this recipe will keep well for a week. For longer-term storage, seal in a freezer-safe container and thaw before use.

PREP TIME: 5 minutes
COOK TIME: 10 minutes

INGREDIENTS | YIELDS 2 CUPS

2 (8-ounce) cans tomato sauce

3 tablespoons apple cider vinegar

2 tablespoons molasses

1 tablespoon honey

1 teaspoon liquid smoke

2 teaspoons onion powder

1½ teaspoons ground cumin

1 teaspoon ground paprika

½ teaspoon garlic powder

½ teaspoon freshly ground black pepper

⅛ teaspoon ground cayenne

1. Combine ingredients in a medium saucepan and simmer over medium-low heat 10 minutes.

2. Remove from heat and pour into a clean lidded jar. Refrigerate and use within a week.

PER 1-TABLESPOON SERVING Calories: 12 | Fat: 0.1 g | Protein: 0.3 g | Sodium: 80 mg | Fiber: 0.3 g | Carbohydrates: 3.0 g | Sugar: 2.4 g

All-Purpose Seasoning

An all-purpose seasoning blend for those who'd rather make their own or have difficulty finding a commercial variety they enjoy, this recipe tastes great on everything from scrambled eggs to pasta, baked potatoes, popcorn, and so much more. Add additional herbs, spices, or dehydrated vegetables if desired. Feel free to double or triple the recipe and store in a large airtight container for convenience.

PREP TIME: 5 minutes
COOK TIME: N/A

INGREDIENTS | YIELDS ½ CUP

3 tablespoons nutritional yeast

1½ tablespoons dried parsley

1 tablespoon onion powder

2½ teaspoons garlic powder

2 teaspoons dried basil

1½ teaspoons dried marjoram

1½ teaspoons ground mustard

1 teaspoon dried dill

1 teaspoon dried oregano

1 teaspoon fennel seeds

1 teaspoon ground paprika

½ teaspoon dried thyme

½ teaspoon ground rosemary

¼ teaspoon ground allspice

¼ teaspoon ground cumin

¼ teaspoon ground sage

1. Place all ingredients in a small food processor or spice grinder and pulse until combined.

2. Store in an airtight container and use within a year.

PER 1-TABLESPOON SERVING Calories: 17 | Fat: 0.2 g | Protein: 1.4 g | Sodium: 4 mg | Fiber: 1.2 g | Carbohydrates: 3.1 g | Sugar: 0.2 g

Chili Seasoning

If you have difficulty finding commercial chili seasoning, make your own! It's quick, affordable, and best yet, the individual seasonings can be adjusted to suit your taste. After assembling the seasoning, store in a tightly sealed container in a cool, dark place. Although it's convenient to keep spices on the counter, it compromises their flavor.

PREP TIME: 5 minutes
COOK TIME: N/A

INGREDIENTS | YIELDS ⅔ CUP

2 tablespoons ground cumin

1 tablespoon ground coriander

2 teaspoons dried oregano

1½ teaspoons ground paprika

½ teaspoon dried red pepper flakes

½ teaspoon garlic powder

½ teaspoon onion powder

¼ teaspoon ground mustard

⅛ teaspoon ground cayenne

1. Measure all ingredients into a small mixing bowl and whisk well to combine.

2. Store seasoning in an airtight container and use within 2 years.

PER 1-TABLESPOON SERVING Calories: 9 | Fat: 0.4 g | Protein: 0.5 g | Sodium: 2 mg | Fiber: 0.7 g | Carbohydrates: 1.6 g | Sugar: 0.1 g

CHAPTER 15

Smoothies, Juices, and Drinks

Vitamin A Super Juice

Don't let its looks deceive you; this green juice is absolutely delicious, with its delightful, sweet taste and garden-fresh scent. Packed with vitamin A, each 6-ounce serving contains almost five times the daily recommended value! This juice is also a great source of vitamin C and manganese.

PREP TIME: 10 minutes
COOK TIME: N/A

INGREDIENTS | YIELDS 2¼ CUPS (THREE 6-OUNCE SERVINGS)

3 medium carrots

½ medium cantaloupe, peeled and seeded

1 medium mango, peeled and pitted

1 medium orange, peeled

2 cups packed fresh baby spinach

2 cups packed chopped fresh kale leaves

1 cup fresh cubed pineapple

1. Process ingredients according to juicer instructions.

2. Stir well to combine. Serve immediately or store in an airtight container, refrigerate, and drink within a day. Shake or stir well before using.

PER 6-OUNCE SERVING Calories: 152 | Fat: 0.6 g | Protein: 3.2 g | Sodium: 68 mg | Fiber: 5.9 g | Carbohydrates: 37.7 g | Sugar: 29.7 g

Vitamin A Facts

Vitamin A is a type of antioxidant found in many foods; the most prevalent form in fruits and vegetables is beta carotene. Vitamin A is essential for good vision, especially at night, as it aids in the formation of pigments that control how well your eyes adjust in the dark. Vitamin A is also critical to the immune system, as it controls the production of white blood cells that fight infection in the body.

Vitamin C Me

Feeling rundown and need a burst of energy stat? Skip the supplement pills and powders and get a natural boost from this heavenly peach-colored concoction. Each 6½-ounce serving contains more than 160 percent of the daily recommended intake of vitamin C, almost half the daily value of vitamin A, and more.

PREP TIME: 10 minutes
COOK TIME: N/A

INGREDIENTS | YIELDS 3¼ CUPS (FIVE 6½-OUNCE SERVINGS)

2 cups fresh cubed pineapple

1 cup fresh strawberries, trimmed

1 medium orange, peeled

1 medium mango, peeled and pitted

1 medium lemon, peeled

½ medium cantaloupe, peeled and seeded

½ medium grapefruit, peeled

1. Process ingredients according to juicer instructions.

2. Stir well to combine. Serve immediately or store in an airtight container, refrigerate, and drink within a day. Shake or stir well before using.

PER 6½-OUNCE SERVING Calories: 117 | Fat: 0.4 g | Protein: 1.9 g | Sodium: 6 mg | Fiber: 4.0 g | Carbohydrates: 30.0 g | Sugar: 24.4 g

Homemade Vegetable Juice

This amazing juice is pure vegetable bliss. This additive-free juice has an appealing orange-red color and light refreshing taste. Delicious on its own, it can also be spiked (think Bloody Mary) or seasoned to taste in a multitude of ways. Use it in lieu of or in combination with broth in any recipe.

PREP TIME: 10 minutes
COOK TIME: N/A

INGREDIENTS | YIELDS 3¾ CUPS (FIVE 6-OUNCE SERVINGS)

3 ripe medium tomatoes

2 medium carrots

2 medium stalks celery

1 medium red bell pepper, seeded

1 medium cucumber, peeled

2 cups packed fresh baby spinach

½ medium onion, peeled

1 lemon, peeled

3 cloves garlic, peeled

¼ cup fresh cilantro

1. Process ingredients according to juicer instructions.

2. Stir well to combine. Serve immediately or store in an airtight container, refrigerate, and drink within a day. Shake or stir well before using.

PER 6-OUNCE SERVING Calories: 46 | Fat: 0.2 g | Protein: 2.1 g | Sodium: 44 mg | Fiber: 3.2 g | Carbohydrates: 10.5 g | Sugar: 5.3 g

Make It Your Own!

Fresh juices and smoothies can be altered easily to correspond with the seasons and personal taste. When trying out completely new flavoring, start small and work your way up, ⅛ teaspoon at a time, until you reach a level you enjoy. Try flavoring this vegetable juice, for instance, with spices such as ground cumin, coriander, cayenne, or black pepper, and a splash of hot sauce or low-sodium soy sauce.

Feed Your Mind Smoothie

This rich, deeply purple-hued smoothie is reminiscent of a frosty peanut butter and jelly sandwich. It's jam-packed with brain-boosting vitamins and nutrients and makes a smart way to start any day. Regular Concord grape juice may be substituted for all or part of the white grape juice if desired. For a thicker, more shake-like smoothie, add a peeled, frozen banana to the mix.

PREP TIME: 5 minutes
COOK TIME: N/A

INGREDIENTS | YIELDS 3 CUPS (FOUR 6-OUNCE SERVINGS)

1 cup frozen blueberries

½ ripe medium avocado, pitted and flesh removed

2 tablespoons peanut butter

1 cup packed fresh baby spinach

1 cup 100% pomegranate juice

1 cup 100% white grape juice

1. Place blueberries, avocado, peanut butter, and spinach in a food processor and pulse to combine. Add fruit juices and pulse until smooth.

2. Serve immediately.

PER 6-OUNCE SERVING Calories: 168 | Fat: 6.5 g | Protein: 2.8 g | Sodium: 49 mg | Fiber: 3.0 g | Carbohydrates: 25.8 g | Sugar: 21.1 g

Juicy Green Zinger

This absolutely delicious, light, and refreshing juice has a great balance of fruit and vegetables, punctuated by a cilantro-ginger-citrus kick. It's chock-full of the good stuff: two times the daily recommended value of vitamin A, and almost a full day's vitamin C, plus vitamins B_6 and E, calcium, copper, folate, iron, magnesium, manganese, and more. It's basically health in a glass, so drink up!

PREP TIME: 10 minutes
COOK TIME: N/A

INGREDIENTS | YIELDS 3½ CUPS (FOUR 7-OUNCE SERVINGS)

2 cups packed fresh baby spinach

2 cups packed chopped fresh kale leaves

1 medium cucumber, peeled

2 medium stalks celery

3 medium apples

1 medium lime, peeled

½ medium ruby red grapefruit, peeled

¼ cup fresh cilantro

1 (1½") piece fresh ginger

1. Process ingredients according to juicer instructions.

2. Stir well to combine. Serve immediately or store in an airtight container, refrigerate, and drink within a day. Shake or stir well before using.

PER 7-OUNCE SERVING Calories: 98 | Fat: 0.2 g | Protein: 2.1 g | Sodium: 31 mg | Fiber: 4.0 g | Carbohydrates: 25.3 g | Sugar: 18.1 g

Blenders and Food Processors and Juicers, Oh My!

Can't decide which appliance to invest in? Think about long-term use. For drinks, a blender is a practical appliance. But if you're looking to chop and purée as well as blend, then a food processor is a better option. Juicers extract the juice from the pulp, thus offering a functionality neither blenders nor food processors possess. Consider how often you will be using the appliance. For light, infrequent use, an inexpensive or compact model works well. For heavy use, invest in a large-capacity appliance with a strong motor and warranty.

Hold-the-Milk Shake

Ripe banana and avocado stand in for dairy in this super-thick and creamy guilt-free green milkshake. It's a delicious treat to enjoy anytime. Filling, yet refreshing, this shake is packed with nutrients, including vitamins A, B_6, C, and E, plus folate, copper, calcium, iron, and more.

PREP TIME: 5 minutes
COOK TIME: N/A

INGREDIENTS | YIELDS 3 CUPS (THREE 8-OUNCE SERVINGS)

2 ripe medium bananas, peeled

½ medium avocado, pitted and flesh removed

1 cup packed fresh baby spinach

2 cups 100% white grape juice

Juice of 1 medium lemon

1. Place bananas, avocado, and spinach in a food processor and pulse to combine. Add fruit juices and pulse until smooth.

2. Serve immediately.

PER 8-OUNCE SERVING Calories: 212 | Fat: 3.4 g | Protein: 2.3 g | Sodium: 18 mg | Fiber: 4.2 g | Carbohydrates: 45.9 g | Sugar: 33.9 g

Sparkling Grapefruit Spritzers

An irresistibly rosy hue and hint of fresh mint make these mocktails a satisfying alternative to champagne. If you only have white grapefruit juice, add a drop of grenadine syrup for a pink color.

PREP TIME: 3 minutes
COOK TIME: N/A

INGREDIENTS | SERVES 4

1 teaspoon chopped fresh mint
1 cup ruby red grapefruit juice
1 (12-ounce) can unflavored seltzer water

1. Divide mint evenly between 4 champagne flutes.

2. Add ¼ cup grapefruit juice to each glass, then top with 3 ounces seltzer.

3. Serve immediately.

PER SERVING Calories: 23 | Fat: 0.0 g | Protein: 0.3 g | Sodium: 11 mg | Fiber: 0.0 g | Carbohydrates: 5.6 g | Sugar: 5.5

Virgin Mimosas

A fabulously fizzy mocktail for buzz-free celebrations, you'll love these Virgin Mimosas. Sparkling white grape juice is sold at most supermarkets and online. For traditional mimosas, substitute a bottle of sparkling wine for the white grape juice. For an added kick to the classic cocktail, add a tablespoon of triple sec to each glass.

PREP TIME: 2 minutes
COOK TIME: N/A

INGREDIENTS | SERVES 8

24 ounces freshly squeezed orange juice
1 (750-ml) bottle sparkling white grape juice

1. Pour 3 ounces orange juice into 8 champagne flutes, then top with 3 ounces sparkling grape juice.

2. Serve immediately.

PER SERVING Calories: 100 | Fat: 0.1 g | Protein: 0.6 g | Sodium: 18 mg | Fiber: 0.2 g | Carbohydrates: 24.5 g | Sugar: 22.0 g

Make Your Own Sparkling Grape Juice!

If you can't find sparkling grape juice locally, make your own at home. All you'll need is a can of frozen white grape juice concentrate and a bottle of plain seltzer water. Refrigerate the juice concentrate and seltzer, removing once the juice is thawed and the seltzer chilled. Reconstitute the juice according to package directions using the seltzer instead of plain water. Stir gently to maximize bubbles. Enjoy!

Ginger Lemonade

There's nothing so refreshing on a hot day as a glass of ice-cold lemonade. In this recipe, the spicy flavor and aroma of fresh ginger adds depth, sophistication, and kick to the beloved classic. Serve immediately or steep in the refrigerator; the longer the lemonade sits, the stronger the ginger becomes.

PREP TIME: 10 minutes
COOK TIME: N/A

INGREDIENTS | SERVES 6

¼ cup minced fresh ginger

Grated zest of 1 medium lemon

½ cup freshly squeezed lemon juice

4 cups water

½ cup agave nectar

Ginger Facts

Ginger is the root of a flowering perennial plant originally native to Asia. It has been used for hundreds of years as a natural remedy for many ailments, particularly nausea. It can be eaten raw, cooked, or ground, and adds a spicy, distinctive flavor to both sweet and savory dishes. Ginger contains antioxidants believed to improve cognitive ability, inhibit cancer, and prevent cardiovascular disease.

1. Place ginger and lemon zest in a pitcher. Add lemon juice, water, and agave and stir well to combine.

2. Place pitcher in refrigerator and allow lemonade to steep or serve immediately.

3. When ready to serve, pour lemonade through a fine-mesh sieve into ice-filled glasses. Serve immediately.

PER SERVING Calories: 87 | Fat: 0.0 g | Protein: 0.2 g | Sodium: 6 mg | Fiber: 1.6 g | Carbohydrates: 23.6 g | Sugar: 20.6 g

Cranberry Limeade

The cranberry juice and lime used in this Cranberry Limeade are a match made in heaven. Sweet, tart, and tangy, this drink is best served ice cold.

PREP TIME: 5 minutes
COOK TIME: N/A

INGREDIENTS | SERVES 4

Grated zest of 1 medium lime
1 cup freshly squeezed lime juice
3 cups water
1 cup cranberry juice (100% juice blend)
¼ cup agave nectar

1. Measure all ingredients into a small pitcher and stir well to combine.

2. Serve immediately over ice or refrigerate and serve within 2 days.

PER SERVING Calories: 104 | Fat: 0.1 g | Protein: 0.5 g | Sodium: 9 mg | Fiber: 1.5 g | Carbohydrates: 29.1 g | Sugar: 23.7 g

Classic Sangria

Delicious and refreshing, this Classic Sangria is perfect for summer get-togethers. An inexpensive, fruity red wine, such as Garnacha (Grenache), Tempranillo, Malbec, Bonarda, or Zinfandel, works best in this recipe.

PREP TIME: 1 hour
COOK TIME: N/A

INGREDIENTS | SERVES 12

1 (1.5-liter) bottle red wine
1 cup triple sec
1 cup lemonade
1 large orange, sliced
1 large lemon, sliced
1 large lime, sliced

1. Pour wine, triple sec, and lemonade into a large pitcher and stir well to combine.

2. Add sliced fruit and stir gently.

3. Refrigerate at least 1 hour before serving. May be refrigerated up to 3 days.

4. Serve over ice and garnish with fruit slices from the pitcher if desired.

PER SERVING Calories: 213 | Fat: 0.0 g | Protein: 0.0 g | Sodium: 0 mg | Fiber: 0.0 g | Carbohydrates: 7.4 g | Sugar: 2.1 g

Mulled Wine

Perfect for winter parties and holiday gatherings, this deliciously steamy, spiked, and spiced combination of red wine and apple cider will keep you and your guests warm and happy. Choose an inexpensive, fruity red wine for this recipe, such as Zinfandel or Merlot.

PREP TIME: 10 minutes
COOK TIME: 15 minutes

INGREDIENTS | SERVES 8

1 (750-ml) bottle red wine

3 cups apple cider

1 cup apple juice

½ cup triple sec

1 medium navel orange, sliced

1 large red apple, cored and diced

¼ cup whole cranberries, rinsed

4 whole cinnamon sticks

2 star anise pods

8 whole cloves

What Is Star Anise?

Star anise are small, brown, star-shaped seed pods that come from a tree native to China. The pods have an anise or black licorice flavor and are used in many types of cooking. The ground pods are one of the components of the classic Chinese five-spice powder. Try adding a star anise pod to your favorite pot of tea or simmer in a stovetop potpourri.

1. Pour wine, apple cider, apple juice, and triple sec into a large stockpot and stir to combine.

2. Add orange, apple, cranberries, cinnamon, star anise, and cloves to the pot and stir gently to combine.

3. Place the stockpot over medium-low heat and simmer, stirring frequently, until mixture begins to lightly steam, 15 minutes. You want to warm the wine, not boil the alcohol off!

4. Remove from heat. Ladle into mugs and garnish with some of the fruit.

5. Serve immediately.

PER SERVING Calories: 284 | Fat: 0.1 g | Protein: 0.2 g | Sodium: 7 mg | Fiber: 0.2 g | Carbohydrates: 20.6 g | Sugar: 13.8 g

Maple Mocha Frappé

A creamy concoction of coffee, cocoa, almond milk, and ripe banana, this makes a great breakfast drink or anytime pick-me-up. The stronger the brewed coffee, the more flavor it lends to the frappé. For a fabulous frozen frappé, peel and freeze the bananas ahead of time.

PREP TIME: 3 minutes
COOK TIME: N/A

INGREDIENTS | SERVES 3

2 ripe medium bananas, peeled
¾ cup brewed coffee, cooled
¾ cup unsweetened almond milk
2 tablespoons pure maple syrup
1 tablespoon unsweetened cocoa powder

1. Place bananas in a food processor and purée.

2. Add remaining ingredients and pulse until smooth and creamy.

3. Serve immediately.

PER SERVING Calories: 116 | Fat: 1.0 g | Protein: 1.5 g | Sodium: 43 mg | Fiber: 2.7 g | Carbohydrates: 28.0 g | Sugar: 17.7 g

Thin Mint Cocoa

This minty drink is heaven in cocoa form. A healthy vegan version of the traditional treat, this recipe will make mouths and tummies tingle.

PREP TIME: 5 minutes
COOK TIME: 5 minutes

INGREDIENTS | SERVES 4

3½ cups vanilla almond milk
¼ cup unsweetened cocoa powder
¼ cup (unpacked) brown sugar
¼ teaspoon peppermint extract

Peppermint Facts

Peppermint is a perennial herb, and its ability to spread and take over a garden is legendary. Its distinctive flavor and tingly freshness enhances drinks, sweets, and salads, as well as many commercial products such as toothpaste. Peppermint is said to soothe upset stomachs, aid with digestion, and protect against cancer.

1. Measure milk into a medium saucepan and place over medium-high heat.

2. Cook until milk begins to steam, roughly 3–5 minutes, then add cocoa and brown sugar and whisk well to combine.

3. Remove from heat. Stir in peppermint extract and serve immediately.

PER SERVING Calories: 126 | Fat: 2.9 g | Protein: 1.9 g | Sodium: 143 mg | Fiber: 2.0 g | Carbohydrates: 26.0 g | Sugar: 22.9 g

Sweet Chai Tea

*Basic black tea, oolong tea, or an herbal tea blend such as orange
or ginger all work wonderfully in this recipe, so feel free to mix
things up! Serve over ice for a refreshing treat in hot weather.*

PREP TIME: 5 minutes
COOK TIME: 5 minutes

INGREDIENTS | SERVES 6

5 cups water

1 cup almond milk

½ cup agave nectar

1 teaspoon vanilla extract

¼ teaspoon ground cloves

¼ teaspoon ground ginger

⅛ teaspoon ground allspice

⅛ teaspoon ground cardamom

⅛ teaspoon ground cinnamon

6 black tea bags, strings removed

1. Place water, milk, agave, vanilla, cloves, ginger, allspice, cardamom, and cinnamon in a large saucepan and whisk until combined. Add tea bags and stir well.

2. Heat over high until contents begin to steam but have not yet boiled, about 5 minutes. Turn off heat and let rest 1 minute.

3. Remove tea bags and ladle into a teapot or mugs. Serve immediately.

PER SERVING Calories: 94 | Fat: 0.4 g | Protein: 0.2 g | Sodium: 26 mg | Fiber: 1.4 g | Carbohydrates: 23.6 g | Sugar: 21.3 g

CHAPTER 16

MIND Diet Desserts

Maple-Carrot Energy Cake

Dense, filling, and subtly sweet, every inch of this cake is packed with raisins, nuts, and carrots. It makes a great hiking snack, power breakfast, or guilt-free dessert and is something to turn to whenever you need a boost of energy without time for a meal. Bake, slice, and freeze this cake in individual zip-top sandwich bags and you have 16 wholesome brain-boosting, body-fueling bars to grab, thaw, and enjoy on the go!

PREP TIME: 15 minutes
COOK TIME: 1 hour

INGREDIENTS | SERVES 16

1 teaspoon plus ¼ cup olive oil, divided

1 tablespoon plus 1 cup unbleached all-purpose flour, divided

¾ cup seedless raisins

1 cup pineapple juice

2 tablespoons ground flaxseed

6 tablespoons water

2 cups grated carrot

½ cup pure maple syrup

¼ cup unsweetened applesauce

1 cup white whole-wheat flour

¼ cup chopped walnuts

1 tablespoon baking powder

1 teaspoon ground cinnamon

½ teaspoon ground allspice

¼ teaspoon ground ginger

⅛ teaspoon ground cloves

White Whole-Wheat Flour

Hard red wheat, the type of flour used in many whole-wheat breads, is high in nutrients, but its flavor can be overpowering. White whole-wheat flour has the same health benefits as red, but with a much lighter taste and texture. It can often be used interchangeably with all-purpose flour, and is a great way of boosting a recipe's fiber and nutrients without compromising taste.

1. Preheat oven to 375°F. Grease and flour an 8" square cake pan using 1 tablespoon olive oil and 1 tablespoon unbleached all-purpose flour and set aside.

2. Place raisins in a small bowl, add pineapple juice, and set aside 10 minutes to soften.

3. Measure flaxseed into a small bowl, add water, and stir to combine. Set aside to thicken.

4. In a large mixing bowl, combine raisins and pineapple juice, carrot, maple syrup, applesauce, and remaining oil.

5. Measure flours, walnuts, baking powder, cinnamon, allspice, ginger, and cloves into another medium mixing bowl and whisk well to combine.

6. Add flour mixture to raisin mixture, then add flaxseed mixture and stir to combine.

7. Pour batter into prepared pan. Place pan on the middle rack in oven and bake until tester inserted into center comes out clean, 50–60 minutes.

8. Remove pan from oven and place on a wire rack to cool to touch. Cut into slices and serve.

PER SERVING Calories: 165 | Fat: 5.3 g | Protein: 2.7 g | Sodium: 103 mg | Fiber: 2.4 g | Carbohydrates: 28.6 g | Sugar: 12.8 g

Sweet Corn Muffins

They're sweet, they're soft, and they're even a little crunchy on top. These cholesterol-free muffins are an amazing dessert that makes any meal—breakfast, lunch, or dinner—better! Best of all? They're table-ready in just 20 minutes!

PREP TIME: 5 minutes
COOK TIME: 15 minutes

INGREDIENTS | YIELDS 1 DOZEN

1 cup cornmeal
1 cup white whole-wheat flour
½ cup sugar
1 tablespoon baking powder
¾ cup almond milk
½ cup olive oil
1 teaspoon vanilla extract

1. Preheat oven to 400°F. Line a 12-muffin tin with paper liners and set aside.

2. Place cornmeal, flour, sugar, and baking powder in a medium mixing bowl and whisk well to combine.

3. Add milk, oil, and vanilla and stir just until combined.

4. Divide batter evenly between muffin cups. Place muffin tin on middle rack in oven and bake 15 minutes, until tester inserted into center of muffin comes clean.

5. Remove from oven and place pan on a wire rack to cool. Cool 10 minutes before removing muffins from pan and placing on wire rack to cool fully.

PER MUFFIN Calories: 187 | Fat: 9.4 g | Protein: 2.2 g | Sodium: 135 mg | Fiber: 2.1 g | Carbohydrates: 24.7 g | Sugar: 8.9 g

Chewy Pumpkin Oatmeal Raisin Cookies

Super chewy and fabulously flavorful, these oatmeal raisin cookies are made even better by the addition of pumpkin! Soft, sweet, and amazingly delicious, you'll find yourself eating them by the handful, so watch out.

PREP TIME: 5 minutes
COOK TIME: 16 minutes

INGREDIENTS | YIELDS 4 DOZEN

1 cup pumpkin purée
1⅔ cups sugar
2 tablespoons molasses
1½ teaspoons vanilla extract
⅔ cup olive oil
1 tablespoon ground flaxseed
2 teaspoons baking soda
1 teaspoon ground cinnamon
½ teaspoon ground nutmeg
1 cup unbleached all-purpose flour
1 cup white whole-wheat flour
1⅓ cups rolled oats
1 cup seedless raisins

1. Preheat oven to 350°F. Line two baking sheets with parchment and set aside.

2. Measure ingredients into a large mixing bowl and stir together using a rubber spatula; scrape the bottom and sides of the bowl to incorporate everything fully.

3. Scoop batter out by tablespoons—a small retractable ice-cream scoop works wonderfully here—and place on the parchment-lined baking sheets.

4. Place sheets on middle rack in oven and bake 16 minutes, until golden brown. Remove from oven and transfer cookies to a wire rack to cool.

5. Repeat process with remaining batter. Store cooled cookies in an airtight container for up to 3 days.

PER 2-COOKIE SERVING Calories: 186 | Fat: 6.5 g | Protein: 2.1 g | Sodium: 106 mg | Fiber: 1.8 g | Carbohydrates: 31.3 g | Sugar: 19.0 g

Grilled Pineapple

Fire up the grill and get ready for a treat! Sweet, juicy pineapple gets even better with heat, transforming into a sophisticated, succulent dessert. It's a healthy and delicious way to end a meal, with almost no effort. For a spicier version, add ⅛ teaspoon ground cayenne to the marinade. This also makes a fabulous fruit-based salsa; try using it in Mango Salsa (Chapter 14).

PREP TIME: 10 minutes
COOK TIME: 10 minutes

INGREDIENTS | SERVES 8

1 fresh ripe whole pineapple
1 tablespoon agave nectar
1 tablespoon lime juice
1 tablespoon olive oil
½ teaspoon ground ginger

1. Heat the grill to medium-high.

2. Cut off the top and bottom of the pineapple. Carefully remove the spiky outer peel, then slice the pineapple in half lengthwise. Slice each half again lengthwise to make 4 quarters. Slice down the center of each quarter to remove the hard inner core. Cut each quarter into 1" slices. Place pineapple in a large mixing bowl.

3. Measure remaining ingredients into a small mixing bowl and whisk well to combine. Add dressing to pineapple and toss well to coat.

4. Place pineapple slices on the grill and cook 5 minutes. Flip slices and grill another 5 minutes, until char marks appear on pineapple.

5. Remove from grill and serve immediately.

PER SERVING Calories: 52 | Fat: 1.7 g | Protein: 0.3 g | Sodium: 0 mg | Fiber: 1.0 g | Carbohydrates: 10.0 g | Sugar: 7.7 g

Curry Cookies

These deliciously different cookies are crisp on the outside and super soft in the middle. The combination of curry powder, peanut butter, and banana may sound strange, but it's so good! For less heat, omit the ground cayenne.

PREP TIME: 10 minutes
COOK TIME: 12 minutes

INGREDIENTS | YIELDS 2½ DOZEN

1 ripe medium banana, peeled and mashed

¾ cup sugar

⅓ cup peanut butter

¼ cup almond milk

3 tablespoons olive oil

1 tablespoon molasses

1 teaspoon vanilla extract

1 cup white whole-wheat flour

2 teaspoons baking powder

1 tablespoon curry powder

½ teaspoon ground ginger

¼ teaspoon ground cardamom

⅛ teaspoon ground cayenne

1. Preheat oven to 350°F. Line two baking sheets with parchment and set aside.

2. Place banana in a medium mixing bowl. Add sugar, peanut butter, milk, oil, molasses, and vanilla and stir well to combine. Add remaining ingredients and stir just until combined. The dough will be very thick and sticky.

3. Drop by tablespoonfuls onto parchment-lined baking sheets. Place sheets on the middle rack in oven and bake 12 minutes, until lightly golden.

4. Remove from oven. Transfer cookies to a wire rack to cool. Store cooled cookies in an airtight container.

PER 2-COOKIE SERVING Calories: 103 | Fat: 0.4 g | Protein: 1.2 g | Sodium: 68 mg | Fiber: 1.5 g | Carbohydrates: 19.6 g | Sugar: 12.2 g

Ice-Cream Scoops Make Perfect Cookies!

Instead of fumbling with tablespoons, scoop out cookie dough using a small retractable ice-cream scoop. Ice-cream scoops produce uniform, picture-perfect cookies and reduce the hassle and mess of working with often thick, sticky doughs and batters. Small scoops are sold in a variety of sizes at kitchenware shops and other retailers as well as online.

Cherry-Blueberry Crisp

This dish is made up of ripe, luscious fruit baked beneath a sweet oatmeal crumb. Use fresh fruit when available and frozen fruit in the off-months. Strawberries or any combination of mixed berries may be substituted for all or part of the cherries and blueberries in this recipe for another delicious crisp.

PREP TIME: 15 minutes
COOK TIME: 30 minutes

INGREDIENTS | SERVES 8

3 cups ripe sweet cherries, pitted
3 cups ripe blueberries, washed
⅓ cup sugar
1 tablespoon lemon juice
1 tablespoon cornstarch
½ cup rolled oats
½ cup white whole-wheat flour
⅓ cup (packed) brown sugar
1 teaspoon ground cinnamon
¼ teaspoon ground allspice
3 tablespoons olive oil
1 tablespoon vanilla extract

1. Preheat oven to 375°F.

2. Place cherries and blueberries in a large mixing bowl. Add sugar, lemon juice, and cornstarch and toss well to combine. Transfer mixture to a 2-quart baking pan and set aside.

3. Measure oats, flour, brown sugar, cinnamon, and allspice into a medium mixing bowl and whisk well to combine. Add oil and vanilla; mix and squeeze with your hands to form a coarse crumb. Sprinkle crumb topping evenly over berries in the pan.

4. Place pan on middle rack in oven and bake 30 minutes, until golden brown.

5. Remove from oven and place on wire rack to cool. Serve warm or cool.

PER SERVING Calories: 233 | Fat: 5.6 g | Protein: 2.7 g | Sodium: 3 mg | Fiber: 4.2 g | Carbohydrates: 45.3 g | Sugar: 30.5 g

Fresh Pear Cake with Cardamom and Pecans

Light, airy, and fragrant, this moist and flavorful cake is sure to be one of your favorites. Try it and you'll see why! This is a perfect recipe for sharing; it's great for parties, potlucks, church, or school events. Apples may be substituted for a portion of the pears; try baking different combinations, with different types of pears and apples, and decide which you like best.

PREP TIME: 15 minutes
COOK TIME: 35 minutes

INGREDIENTS | SERVES 16

1 teaspoon plus ½ cup olive oil, divided

1 tablespoon plus 1 cup unbleached all-purpose flour, divided

3 medium fresh pears, peeled, cored, and chopped

⅔ cup sugar

2 tablespoons lemon juice

1 tablespoon ground flaxseed

3 tablespoons water

¼ cup white whole-wheat flour

1 tablespoon baking powder

½ teaspoon ground cardamom

¼ cup chopped pecans

1½ teaspoons almond extract

1½ teaspoons vanilla extract

Pear Facts

Pears are native to Eurasia and have been cultivated since Roman times. Eaten raw, cooked, and dried, pears are also prized for their delicious juice, which can be fermented into an alcoholic cider. Not all pear varieties have the traditional "pear" shape; some are round like apples. When enjoying fresh pears, wash and consume without peeling; the skin contains important phytonutrients and fiber. Unripe pears should be stored at room temperature; once ripe, they should be refrigerated. Test for ripeness by pressing gently around the stem and neck; ripe, juicy pears will yield to gentle pressure.

1. Preheat oven to 375°F. Grease and flour an 8" square baking pan with 1 teaspoon olive oil and 1 teaspoon unbleached all-purpose flour and set aside.

2. Place pears, sugar, and lemon juice in a medium mixing bowl and stir to combine. Set aside.

3. Measure flaxseed and water into a small bowl and stir to combine. Set aside to thicken.

4. Measure flours, baking powder, cardamom, and pecans into a clean medium mixing bowl and whisk well to combine.

5. Add flaxseed mixture, remaining oil, almond, and vanilla to pears and stir well. Add flour mixture to pears and stir until combined. The batter will be very thick and sticky.

6. Pour batter into prepared pan and spread to even. Place pan on middle rack in oven and bake 35 minutes, until golden brown.

7. Remove pan from oven and place on a wire rack to cool. Slice into squares and serve.

PER SERVING Calories: 164 | Fat: 8.3 g | Protein: 1.5 g | Sodium: 92 mg | Fiber: 1.6 g | Carbohydrates: 20.8 g | Sugar: 11.0 g

Chocolate Gingerbread

This amazingly moist, cocoa-spiked gingerbread is simply delicious. If caffeine is an issue for you, use an equal amount of decaffeinated coffee for the traditional brew. If you don't have crystallized ginger on hand, substitute chocolate chips, raisins, or chopped dried fruit instead.

PREP TIME: 10 minutes
COOK TIME: 30 minutes

INGREDIENTS | SERVES 16

1 teaspoon plus ½ cup olive oil, divided
⅓ cup unsweetened cocoa powder
⅔ cup unbleached all-purpose flour
⅔ cup white whole-wheat flour
1 cup (packed) brown sugar
2 teaspoons baking powder
2½ teaspoons ground ginger
1 teaspoon ground cinnamon
1 cup brewed coffee, cooled to room temperature
¼ cup chopped crystallized ginger
2 tablespoons apple cider vinegar

1. Preheat oven to 375°F. Lightly oil an 8" square baking pan with 1 teaspoon olive oil and dust with a tiny amount of flour or cocoa powder. Set aside.

2. Measure the cocoa powder, flours, sugar, baking powder, ground ginger, and cinnamon into a medium mixing bowl and whisk well to combine. Add the coffee, ½ cup oil, crystallized ginger, and vinegar and stir just until combined.

3. Pour batter into prepared pan. Place pan on middle rack in oven and bake 30 minutes, until tester inserted in center comes clean.

4. Remove pan from oven and place on wire rack to cool. Slice into squares and serve.

PER SERVING Calories: 158 | Fat: 7.2 g | Protein: 1.6 g | Sodium: 66 mg | Fiber: 1.6 g | Carbohydrates: 23.4 g | Sugar: 13.9 g

Peanut Butter Chocolate Chip Blondies

Peanut butter and chocolate make a mouthwatering combination in these chewy cookie bars. For extra crunch, sprinkle a tablespoon of chopped unsalted peanuts on top of the batter before baking. For brownie bars, reduce the unbleached flour to ¼ cup and add ¼ cup unsweetened cocoa powder.

PREP TIME: 10 minutes
COOK TIME: 35 minutes

INGREDIENTS | SERVES 16

1 teaspoon plus 6 tablespoons olive oil, divided
½ cup unbleached all-purpose flour
½ cup white whole-wheat flour
1 cup quick oats
½ cup brown sugar
½ cup sugar
2 teaspoons baking powder
½ cup peanut butter
½ cup almond milk
1 tablespoon vanilla extract
½ cup semisweet chocolate chips

1. Preheat oven to 350°F. Lightly oil an 8" square baking pan with 1 teaspoon olive oil and set aside.

2. Measure flours, oats, sugars, and baking powder into a medium mixing bowl and whisk well to combine. Add remaining ingredients and stir well to combine. Press batter into the prepared pan.

3. Place pan on middle rack in oven and bake 35 minutes, until golden brown.

4. Remove from oven and place on wire rack to cool fully. Cut into bars and serve.

PER SERVING Calories: 181 | Fat: 10.0 g | Protein: 3.5 g | Sodium: 103 mg | Fiber: 1.7 g | Carbohydrates: 19.6 g | Sugar: 9.0 g

Cookie Baking Tip

When baking cookie bars, allow them to fully cool in the pan before slicing and removing. This keeps the edges intact and helps ensure your cookie bars look picture-perfect. To get evenly sized bars, slice half-way through the pan, then divide each half in half and slice again.

Lemon Cookies

Crisp, buttery, yet cholesterol-free, these deliciously simple cookies shine with bright citrus flavor. If you don't have fresh lemons, use ½ cup bottled lemon juice and ½ teaspoon lemon extract instead. Substitute lime, orange, or grapefruit juice for a different twist on the same recipe.

PREP TIME: 5 minutes
COOK TIME: 10 minutes

INGREDIENTS | YIELDS 3 DOZEN

1½ cups unbleached all-purpose flour
1 cup white whole-wheat flour
1½ cups sugar
1 tablespoon baking powder
¾ cup olive oil
Juice and grated zest of 2 large lemons
1 tablespoon vanilla extract

1. Preheat oven to 350°F. Get out two baking sheets and set aside.

2. Measure flours, sugar, and baking powder into a medium mixing bowl and whisk well to combine. Add remaining ingredients and stir to form a stiff dough.

3. Drop by rounded tablespoons onto the ungreased baking sheets. Place sheets on middle rack in oven and bake 10 minutes, until cookies are pale and have spread out.

4. Remove from oven, cool on baking sheets a few minutes, then transfer to a wire rack to cool fully.

5. Serve cooled cookies or store in an airtight container for up to 3 days.

PER COOKIE Calories: 103 | Fat: 4.5 g | Protein: 1.0 g | Sodium: 40 mg | Fiber: 0.6 g | Carbohydrates: 15.1 g | Sugar: 8.4 g

Whole-Grain Strawberry Bread

A fabulous, fruit-filled quick bread, this Whole-Grain Strawberry Bread is summer fresh! It's moist with juicy bits of strawberry and has an irresistible cinnamon scent. Spread with peanut butter for a delicious PBJ sandwich—no jelly needed

PREP TIME: 10 minutes
COOK TIME: 1 hour

INGREDIENTS | SERVES 16

1 teaspoon plus ⅔ cup olive oil, divided
1 cup unbleached all-purpose flour
½ cup white whole-wheat flour
1¼ cups mashed strawberries
¾ cup sugar
2 large eggs, beaten
2 teaspoons ground cinnamon
1 teaspoon baking soda

Cut the Fat!

When looking to minimize oil in baked goods, try substituting unsweetened applesauce, mashed banana, or puréed prunes for all or part of the fat. When sautéing, coat the bottom of pans with water or broth. Little steps like these add up, and will keep you slimmer and healthier.

1. Preheat oven to 350°F. Grease an 8" loaf pan with 1 teaspoon olive oil and set aside.

2. Measure all ingredients into a large mixing bowl and stir just until combined. Pour batter into the prepared loaf pan.

3. Place pan on middle rack in oven and bake 1 hour, until tester inserted in center comes clean.

4. Remove from oven and place pan on a wire rack to cool. Serve warm or at room temperature.

PER SERVING Calories: 174 | Fat: 9.7 g | Protein: 2.2 g | Sodium: 9 mg | Fiber: 1.3 g | Carbohydrates: 19.9 g | Sugar: 10.3 g

Oven-Baked Apple Pancake

Moist, airy, and delicious, this homey dessert will impress with its taste and simplicity. The oven does all the work; just whisk together the ingredients, pour, and bake. In just 30 minutes, you've got a healthy, heavenly treat. For variety, substitute diced pears, plums, or peaches for the apple, or add chopped nuts or dried fruit to the batter. Serve for breakfast or brunch, too!

PREP TIME: 5 minutes
COOK TIME: 25 minutes

INGREDIENTS | SERVES 8

1 teaspoon olive oil
2 cups peeled, cored, and diced apple
1 tablespoon vanilla extract
1 tablespoon baking powder
½ cup unbleached all-purpose flour
½ cup white whole-wheat flour
⅓ cup unsweetened applesauce
⅓ cup plus ¼ cup (for drizzling) pure maple syrup, divided
¾ cup almond milk
1 tablespoon sugar
½ teaspoon ground cinnamon

1. Preheat oven to 400°F. Lightly oil a large ovenproof skillet with 1 teaspoon olive oil and set aside.

2. Place apple, vanilla, baking powder, flours, applesauce, ⅓ cup maple syrup, and milk in a medium mixing bowl and whisk well to combine. Pour batter into the prepared pan and smooth top to even.

3. Combine sugar and cinnamon in a small bowl and sprinkle evenly over the batter.

4. Place pan on middle rack in oven and bake 25 minutes, until golden brown.

5. Remove skillet from oven. Use a rubber spatula and carefully loosen pancake from pan. Slice like a pizza into 8 pieces, drizzle with remaining maple syrup, and serve immediately.

PER SERVING Calories: 156 | Fat: 1.0 g | Protein: 2.1 g | Sodium: 18 mg | Fiber: 1.9 g | Carbohydrates: 35.5 g | Sugar: 20.8 g

Jam-Filled Cupcakes

These light and fluffy cupcakes make eating on the MIND diet fun. The jam keeps them moist, so there's no need to frost. Add ½ teaspoon lemon, orange, or maple extract instead of the almond, and play around with different jams to find your favorite flavor combinations. For chocolate cupcakes, add ⅓ cup unsweetened cocoa powder and reduce the all-purpose flour to ¾ cup.

PREP TIME: 10 minutes
COOK TIME: 22 minutes

INGREDIENTS | YIELDS 1 DOZEN

⅔ cup almond milk
½ teaspoon apple cider vinegar
⅔ cup agave nectar
⅓ cup olive oil
1½ teaspoons vanilla extract
½ teaspoon almond extract
1 cup unbleached all-purpose flour
⅓ cup white whole-wheat flour
1 tablespoon baking powder
¼ cup strawberry jam, at room temperature

Desserts and the MIND Diet

People often equate dieting with deprivation, but sweets can be part of a healthy lifestyle when chosen wisely and consumed in moderation. If you're someone with an above-average sweet tooth, try to channel cravings into the healthy realm of fruit. Keep an array of fresh produce out on the counter and you'll find yourself reaching for it daily. Dried fruit, applesauce, and juice-sweetened fruit cups also make great guilt-free snacks.

1. Preheat oven to 325°F. Line a 12-muffin tin with paper liners and set aside.

2. Place milk and vinegar in a medium mixing bowl. Stir well and set aside 5 minutes to curdle.

3. Add agave, oil, and extracts to milk-vinegar mixture and stir well to combine. Add flours and baking powder and whisk until smooth.

4. Fill each muffin cup with 2 tablespoons batter, top with 1 teaspoon jam, then cover with another 2 tablespoons batter. Try to get the jam in the center of the muffin cup so it's not creeping out to the sides, and be sure to cover the jam completely.

5. Place muffin tin on middle rack in oven and bake 22 minutes, until golden brown.

6. Remove tin from oven and place on wire rack to cool before serving. Cool 10 minutes, then carefully remove cupcakes from tin and place on wire rack to cool fully.

PER SERVING Calories: 178 | Fat: 6.1 g | Protein: 1.6 g | Sodium: 133 mg | Fiber: 1.7 g | Carbohydrates: 30.1 g | Sugar: 17.0 g

Chocolate-Covered Strawberries

These elegant treats are so easy to make at home, you'll never buy them again. Chocolate-covered strawberries are a classic favorite; substitute an equal amount of another fresh or dried fruit, from sliced banana to dried apricots, if desired. For an extra-fancy treat, sprinkle the freshly dipped strawberries with colored sugar or sprinkles, or drizzle with melted white chocolate. If you don't have a microwave, place the chocolate chips and oil into a double boiler and gently melt over low heat, stirring constantly.

PREP TIME: 15 minutes
COOK TIME: 1 minute

INGREDIENTS | SERVES 8

¾ cup semisweet chocolate chips
1 tablespoon olive oil
16 ounces fresh strawberries, washed and dried

1. Line a baking sheet or tray with waxed paper; set aside.

2. Place chocolate chips and oil in a small microwave-safe bowl or mug. Microwave 1 minute, then remove and stir constantly until chocolate is fully melted and smooth.

3. Dip each strawberry into chocolate, then place on the waxed paper. Let strawberries rest at least 10 minutes to harden. Strawberries may be refrigerated and are best consumed within a day.

PER SERVING Calories: 63 | Fat: 3.3 g | Protein: 0.8 g | Sodium: 4 mg | Fiber: 1.5 g | Carbohydrates: 8.1 g | Sugar: 6.2 g

Mango Crumble

Sink your teeth into tender chunks of mango and a cinnamon-scented crust with this MIND diet favorite! For a juicier filling, omit the cornstarch. Can't find mangoes? Substitute 4 cups fresh or canned pineapple chunks, peaches, blueberries, strawberries, or another favorite fruit instead. This is delicious served warm or cool.

PREP TIME: 10 minutes
COOK TIME: 25 minutes

INGREDIENTS | SERVES 8

2 large mangoes, peeled, cored, and cut into 1" chunks

2 tablespoons brown sugar

1 tablespoon cornstarch

1½ teaspoons minced fresh ginger

½ cup unbleached all-purpose flour

½ cup white whole-wheat flour

½ cup sugar

1 teaspoon ground cinnamon

½ teaspoon ground ginger

3 tablespoons olive oil

1. Preheat oven to 375°F. Get out an 8" square baking pan and set aside.

2. Place mangoes, brown sugar, cornstarch, and fresh ginger in a medium mixing bowl and toss well to coat. Turn mixture out into the baking pan and spread to even.

3. In another medium bowl, whisk together flours, sugar, cinnamon, and ground ginger. Add oil and squeeze the mixture with your hands to form a coarse sand-like crumb. Sprinkle mixture evenly over fruit.

4. Place pan on middle rack in oven and bake 25 minutes until fruit is tender.

5. Remove from oven and place on wire rack to cool. Serve warm or cool.

PER SERVING Calories: 215 | Fat: 5.4 g | Protein: 2.5 g | Sodium: 1 mg | Fiber: 2.8 g | Carbohydrates: 41.5 g | Sugar: 27.3 g

Peppermint Watermelon Granita

Delightfully tingly, this refreshing dessert is the perfect end to a summer meal. To serve, scoop into glasses or bowls and garnish with fresh mint leaves and extra cubed watermelon. Play around with the basic recipe using different flavors of tea or juice and fruit; making your own water ice is fun and easy!

PREP TIME: 2–3 hours
COOK TIME: N/A

INGREDIENTS | SERVES 6

3 peppermint tea bags
3 cups boiling water
3 cups cubed fresh watermelon
1 tablespoon agave nectar

Watermelon Facts

Watermelon is closely related to ground melons and squash. It's low in fat, a good source of fiber, and as its name suggests, one of the juiciest fruits around. Watermelon contains high levels of vitamins A and C as well as lycopene, a cancer-fighting antioxidant. To select a perfectly ripe watermelon, hold it close to your body and thump firmly. If it sounds and feels hollow, it's a keeper. Put back any watermelons without reverb; they tend to be mealy.

1. Place tea bags in a heatproof pitcher or teapot. Add boiling water and steep 5 minutes.

2. Place cubed watermelon in a food processor and purée.

3. Remove tea bags and pour liquid into a 9" × 13" freezer-safe pan.

4. Add watermelon and agave and stir to combine. Cover tightly with plastic wrap and place in freezer.

5. Freeze 2–3 hours, until semi-solid. Remove from freezer and scrape mixture into glasses or bowls. Serve immediately.

PER SERVING Calories: 33 | Fat: 0.1 g | Protein: 0.5 g | Sodium: 0 mg | Fiber: 0.5 g | Carbohydrates: 8.5 g | Sugar: 7.3 g

Homemade Banana Ice Cream

This dessert contains only one ingredient: bananas! Yet when frozen and puréed, the crystallized fruit so perfectly mimics the look, taste, and texture of soft-serve ice cream that it's almost magic. Peel the bananas before freezing to make this the easiest dessert ever. And for an even tastier treat, see the sidebar to learn how to top your Homemade Banana Ice Cream with your very own homemade chocolate shell!

PREP TIME: 2 minutes
COOK TIME: N/A

INGREDIENTS | SERVES 4

4 medium ripe bananas

Homemade Chocolate Shell

If you love the taste and texture of that magical chocolate shell sold in stores and ice-cream parlors, here's how to make your own at home. Simply measure ½ cup chocolate chips into a microwave-safe bowl or mug, add 1 teaspoon olive oil, and microwave for 1 minute. Stir until smooth and drizzle over your favorite frozen dessert. It hardens almost instantly, like magic!

1. Peel bananas, place in a large zip-top plastic bag, and place in freezer. Freeze until solid.

2. Remove bananas from freezer and slice into chunks. Place chunks in a food processor and pulse until smooth.

3. Scoop mixture out and serve immediately.

PER SERVING Calories: 105 | Fat: 0.3 g | Protein: 1.3 g | Sodium: 1 mg | Fiber: 3.1 g | Carbohydrates: 27.0 g | Sugar: 14.4 g

CHAPTER 17

Occasional Foods

Slow Cooker Pot Roast

Pop all of the ingredients into the cooker at 9 A.M. and by 5 P.M. you'll have a meal fit for royalty. The slow cooking renders the vegetables toothsome and the beef tender, which is just what you want when you decide to splurge and have some red meat. Serve each portion with a generous spoonful of the delicious herb-infused broth and partner this dish with sautéed dark leafy greens.

PREP TIME: 10 minutes
COOK TIME: 8 hours

INGREDIENTS | SERVES 8

2 cups beef broth
1 cup red wine
3 cloves garlic, minced
1 teaspoon freshly ground black pepper
1 teaspoon ground mustard
½ teaspoon celery seed
½ teaspoon dried basil
½ teaspoon dried marjoram
½ teaspoon dried oregano
½ teaspoon dried savory
3 medium potatoes, peeled and diced
3 medium carrots, peeled and sliced
1 medium onion, peeled and diced
3½ pounds beef bottom round roast

1. Set slow cooker to medium. Pour in broth, wine, garlic, pepper, mustard, celery seed, basil, marjoram, oregano, and savory and stir to combine. Add potatoes, carrots, and onion and stir. Last, place roast into the pot and flip several times to moisten.

2. Place lid on cooker and simmer 8 hours; turn roast several times if possible. By the end of cooking time, meat will easily pull apart and vegetables will be fork tender.

3. Plate beef with vegetables and broth. Serve immediately.

PER SERVING Calories: 375 | Fat: 8.3 g | Protein: 46.7 g | Sodium: 354 mg | Fiber: 1.9 g | Carbohydrates: 16.5 g | Sugar: 2.2 g

Spaghetti Bolognese

In this recipe, ground beef, sautéed vegetables, tomatoes, herbs, and wine come together in a thick, rich sauce. Substitute your choice of whole-grain pasta for the spaghetti if desired. Serve with a nice Chianti and a big green salad for a classic Italian meal.

PREP TIME: 10 minutes
COOK TIME: 35 minutes

INGREDIENTS | SERVES 6

1 (12-ounce) package whole-grain spaghetti

2 tablespoons olive oil

1 medium onion, peeled and diced

2 medium stalks celery, trimmed and chopped

2 medium carrots, peeled and chopped

3 cloves garlic, minced

1½ pounds extra-lean ground beef

1 (15-ounce) can no salt added diced tomatoes, with juice

2 (8-ounce) cans tomato sauce

⅓ cup red wine

1 tablespoon balsamic vinegar

1 tablespoon agave nectar

1 teaspoon dried basil

½ teaspoon dried marjoram

½ teaspoon dried oregano

½ teaspoon dried thyme

½ teaspoon freshly ground black pepper

½ teaspoon dried red pepper flakes

1. Cook pasta according to package directions. Drain and set aside.

2. Heat oil in a large skillet or sauté pan over medium heat. Add onion and cook, stirring, 2 minutes, until fragrant. Add celery, carrots, and garlic and cook, stirring, 3 minutes until they begin to sweat. Add beef and sauté until browned and cooked through, 5 minutes. Add remaining ingredients and stir well to combine. Cook until mixture begins to bubble, then reduce heat to low, cover, and simmer 25 minutes, stirring occasionally, until thick and bubbly.

3. Remove from heat and spoon over spaghetti. Serve immediately.

PER SERVING Calories: 447 | Fat: 9.3 g | Protein: 34.1 g | Sodium: 497 mg | Fiber: 9.8 g | Carbohydrates: 57.0 g | Sugar: 11.8 g

Cut the Fat

When choosing ground beef or other meats, always buy the leanest cuts possible. When you compare fat for a 4-ounce serving of ground beef, for instance, you can cut your fat intake in half simply by opting for the slightly more expensive 95% lean (5.6 g fat) over the 90% lean (11 g fat). Leaner meat may be more expensive, but better health is worth the small investment.

Seared Sirloin Steaks with Garlicky Greens

Incredibly easy and immensely flavorful, this recipe is worthy of celebration. The meat is juicy, perfectly tender, and medium rare; the greens are amazingly delicious, tart, and garlicky with a mustard tang. Substitute an equal amount of another dark leafy green for the fresh kale if desired. Serve with roasted potatoes and fresh corn for a truly delectable meal.

PREP TIME: 15 minutes
COOK TIME: 25 minutes

INGREDIENTS | SERVES 6

1½ pounds sirloin steak, 1" thick

1½ teaspoons coarsely chopped dried rosemary

½ teaspoon freshly ground black pepper, divided

¼ cup olive oil, divided

¾ cup red wine

4 cloves garlic, minced

2 tablespoons balsamic vinegar

1 teaspoon agave nectar

½ teaspoon mustard

1½ pounds chopped fresh kale leaves, thick stems removed

1. Preheat oven to 400°F. Get out a sided baking sheet and set aside.

2. Trim cut steak into 6 equal portions. Sprinkle steaks with rosemary and ¼ teaspoon pepper.

3. Heat 1 tablespoon oil in a large skillet or sauté pan over medium-high heat. Arrange steaks in the skillet in a single layer (might require two batches) and cook 3–4 minutes per side until nicely browned; only turn steaks once.

4. Remove the skillet from the heat, transfer steaks to the baking sheet, and roast 4–6 minutes more until medium rare. Remove from oven and set aside to rest.

5. Return the skillet to medium-high heat. Carefully add wine, scrape up any browned bits with a wooden spoon, and cook 3–4 minutes until reduced by about half. Add garlic and cook until fragrant, about 10 seconds. Whisk in vinegar, agave, mustard, and remaining ¼ teaspoon pepper. Drizzle in remaining 3 tablespoons oil while whisking constantly.

6. Add the kale and cook, tossing, until leaves are wilted enough to fit comfortably in the skillet, about 2 minutes. Cover the skillet and cook, tossing once or twice, about 5 minutes until just tender.

7. Transfer steaks to plates and top with greens. Serve immediately.

PER SERVING Calories: 399 | Fat: 21.9 g | Protein: 28.1 g | Sodium: 109 mg | Fiber: 4.4 g | Carbohydrates: 13.5 g | Sugar: 4.4 g

Cajun-Style Dirty Rice

This classic Cajun dish has been reworked to be much lower in fat, but it retains all the flavor of the original. It makes a wonderful one-skillet supper or side. Serve with mixed sautéed vegetables and Sweet Corn Muffins (Chapter 16) for a complete and satisfying meal.

PREP TIME: 5 minutes
COOK TIME: 25 minutes

INGREDIENTS | SERVES 4

½ pound extra-lean ground beef

1 large onion, peeled and diced

2 medium stalks celery, trimmed and diced

2 cloves garlic, minced

1 medium bell pepper, seeded and diced

1 cup beef broth

2 teaspoons Worcestershire sauce

1½ teaspoons dried thyme

1 teaspoon dried basil

½ teaspoon dried marjoram

¼ teaspoon freshly ground black pepper

⅛ teaspoon ground cayenne

2 scallions, sliced

3 cups cooked brown rice

1. Place ground beef, onion, celery, and garlic in a medium sauté pan over medium heat. Cook until beef is browned, roughly 5 minutes.

2. Add bell pepper, beef broth, Worcestershire sauce, thyme, basil, marjoram, black pepper, and cayenne and stir to combine. Bring to a boil, then reduce heat to low, cover, and simmer 20 minutes until tender.

3. Remove from heat and stir in scallions. Add cooked rice and stir well to combine. Serve immediately.

PER SERVING Calories: 258 | Fat: 2.9 g | Protein: 17.4 g | Sodium: 308 mg | Fiber: 4.2 g | Carbohydrates: 40.5 g | Sugar: 2.6 g

Pan-Fried Chicken Cutlets with Broccoli Rabe

In this dish, moist and juicy chicken cutlets with a golden breaded crunch are topped with pasta sauce and a sprinkle of Parmesan. It's an irresistible meal. Blanching removes most of the bitterness of the broccoli rabe, so you can really dig in and enjoy. Prepackaged, skinless, boneless, thin-sliced chicken breasts make this a snap to prepare.

PREP TIME: 15 minutes
COOK TIME: 32 minutes

INGREDIENTS | SERVES 6

1½ pounds fresh broccoli rabe, washed and cut into 2" pieces

¼ cup unbleached all-purpose flour

¼ cup white whole-wheat flour

1 large egg

2 tablespoons low-fat milk

1⅓ cups bread crumbs

1½ pounds boneless, skinless, thin-sliced chicken breasts

2 cups (for frying) plus 1 tablespoon (for broccoli rabe) olive oil, divided

3 garlic cloves, minced

¼ teaspoon dried red pepper flakes

¼ teaspoon freshly ground black pepper

1½ cups pasta sauce, divided

6 tablespoons grated Parmesan cheese, divided

1. Place a large stockpot of water over high heat and bring to a boil. Add broccoli rabe to boiling water and cook uncovered 4–5 minutes until tender. Drain in a colander and set aside.

2. Get out three shallow bowls. Measure flours into one and whisk to combine. Beat egg and milk in the second. Place bread crumbs in the third. Dredge each chicken cutlet first in flour, then in egg, then coat thoroughly with bread crumbs. Set breaded cutlet aside on a piece of waxed paper and repeat process until all chicken cutlets are coated.

3. Heat 2 cups oil in a large skillet or sauté pan over medium heat. Place cutlets in hot oil two at a time and fry until golden brown on both sides, 2–4 minutes per side. Remove from oil and place on paper towels to drain. Repeat for remaining cutlets.

4. Heat 1 tablespoon oil in a medium skillet over medium heat. Add garlic and sauté 1 minute, then add broccoli rabe, red pepper flakes, and black pepper and cook, stirring, until warmed through, 1–2 minutes.

5. Remove from heat. Plate cutlets and top with broccoli rabe. Garnish each cutlet with ¼ cup pasta sauce and 1 tablespoon Parmesan. Serve immediately.

PER SERVING Calories: 486 | Fat: 25.0 g | Protein: 36.3 g | Sodium: 619 mg | Fiber: 5.9 g | Carbohydrates: 27.8 g | Sugar: 5.2 g

Crispy Pork Medallions with Apple-Horseradish Sauce

*Looking for an easy, gourmet meal to make any celebration more memorable?
Look no further! Crispy, panko-coated pork is partnered with an absolutely
stupendous sauce. The flavors of apple and pork meld so fluidly; add the
bite of sour cream and kick of horseradish, and it's out of this world!*

PREP TIME: 10 minutes
COOK TIME: 8 minutes

INGREDIENTS | SERVES 4

1 cup unsweetened applesauce

¼ cup fat-free sour cream

3 tablespoons horseradish, excess vinegar squeezed out

2 large eggs

1 cup plain panko bread crumbs

½ teaspoon ground sage

½ teaspoon dried thyme

4 (4-ounce, ½"-thick) boneless pork loin medallions

¼ teaspoon freshly ground black pepper

3 tablespoons olive oil

Pork Facts

Lean pork is considered a healthy meat, especially when consumed in moderation. It contains roughly the same amount of cholesterol per serving as chicken and turkey. Pork is an excellent source of protein, vitamins B_6 and B_{12}, and minerals. Its mild flavor is a great partner to most types of fruit, both fresh and dried. As a lean meat, pork can dry out quickly, so it's important not to overcook.

1. Measure applesauce, sour cream, and horseradish into a small mixing bowl and stir well to combine. Set aside.

2. Beat eggs in a shallow bowl.

3. Measure panko into a second shallow bowl, add sage and thyme, and mix to combine.

4. Lightly season pork with pepper.

5. Dip each loin in egg, then gently press into panko mixture; coat thoroughly.

6. Heat oil in a large skillet or sauté pan over medium heat. Add medallions to hot oil and cook until golden and crispy on bottom, 4 minutes. Flip medallions and repeat on second side, 3–4 minutes.

7. Remove pork from pan, garnish with sauce, and serve immediately.

PER SERVING Calories: 346 | Fat: 16.3 g | Protein: 30.6 g | Sodium: 169 mg | Fiber: 1.2 g | Carbohydrates: 12.0 g | Sugar: 7.1 g

Homemade Pork Sausage Patties

These delicious homemade sausage patties are scented with sage and have a nice red pepper kick. Everyone who tastes them raves about their flavor and simplicity. Some even swear they'll never buy premade breakfast sausage again! High praise indeed.

PREP TIME: 10 minutes
COOK TIME: 10 minutes

INGREDIENTS | SERVES 8

2 pounds lean ground pork
1 large egg white
2 teaspoons brown sugar
2½ teaspoons ground sage
1 teaspoon dried marjoram
¾ teaspoon dried red pepper flakes
½ teaspoon freshly ground black pepper
¼ teaspoon ground rosemary

Get Creative!

Homemade sausage isn't simply for breakfast. Sausage makes a terrific topping for pizza, adds spice and interest to plain pasta and sauce, and elevates boring meatloaf to something special. Double the batch whenever you make sausage, and freeze leftovers for use in future recipes.

1. Combine ingredients in a large bowl and mix well using a fork or your hands. Form mixture into 16 (2") patties.

2. Heat griddle or skillet over medium heat and brown patties on both sides, about 5 minutes per side. Lower heat to medium-low or low if they seem to be burning. Drain on paper towels and serve.

PER SERVING Calories: 144 | Fat: 4.5 g | Protein: 24.4 g | Sodium: 82 mg | Fiber: 0.2 g | Carbohydrates: 1.7 g | Sugar: 1.2 g

Scallops Fra Diavolo

These rich and meaty scallops are simply sublime. Serve over cooked brown rice, quinoa, or whole-grain pasta for a hearty, healthy meal. Fresh or frozen (thawed) scallops work well in this recipe.

PREP TIME: 5 minutes
COOK TIME: 32 minutes

INGREDIENTS | SERVES 4

2 tablespoons olive oil

1 large onion, peeled and chopped

1 medium green bell pepper, seeded and chopped

4 cloves garlic, minced

¼ cup red wine

1 (28-ounce) can stewed tomatoes

1 teaspoon agave nectar

¼ teaspoon dried red pepper flakes

1 pound sea scallops

1. Heat oil in a large skillet or sauté pan over medium heat. Add onion and bell pepper and cook, stirring occasionally, 5 minutes. Add garlic and cook 1 minute. Add wine and cook 1 minute.

2. Stir in tomatoes, agave, and red pepper flakes and bring to a boil. Reduce heat to medium-low and simmer uncovered 15 minutes until sauce begins to thicken. Stir occasionally. If sauce begins to pop and splatter, lower heat further.

3. Add scallops and cook 5–10 minutes until opaque.

4. Remove from heat and serve immediately.

PER SERVING Calories: 242 | Fat: 9.3 g | Protein: 16.1 g | Sodium: 849 mg | Fiber: 2.4 g | Carbohydrates: 20.9 g | Sugar: 12.5 g

Salmon with Mango and Chickpea Salad

The vibrant colors and flavors of this delicious entrée play hopscotch with the senses. The salmon is baked, leaving it delectably crisp on the outside and juicy within, and it is served with a zesty, sweet, and savory salad. If you don't have any fresh mango, substitute another fruit instead, like cubed Grilled Pineapple (Chapter 16).

PREP TIME: 1 hour 10 minutes
COOK TIME: 14 minutes

INGREDIENTS | SERVES 4

2 ripe mangoes, peeled, cored, and diced

1 small red onion, peeled and diced

2 cloves garlic, minced

1 (15-ounce) can chickpeas, drained and rinsed

3 tablespoons chopped fresh cilantro

Juice of 1 medium lime

4 tablespoons olive oil, divided

1 tablespoon agave nectar

½ teaspoon freshly ground black pepper, divided

1 pound fresh salmon, cut into 4 (4-ounce) portions

1 tablespoon lemon juice

½ teaspoon dried dill

1. Place mango, onion, garlic, chickpeas, and cilantro in a medium mixing bowl and toss to combine. Measure lime juice, 2 tablespoons olive oil, agave, and ¼ teaspoon pepper into a small mixing bowl and whisk well. Pour dressing over mango salad and toss to coat. Cover and refrigerate 1 hour to allow the flavors to mingle and develop.

2. Preheat oven to 425°F. Place salmon fillets in a baking dish. Brush with remaining olive oil. Sprinkle with lemon juice, dill, and remaining ¼ teaspoon pepper.

3. Place baking pan on middle rack in oven and bake 12–14 minutes until salmon is opaque.

4. Remove from oven and serve immediately with mango and chickpea salad.

PER SERVING Calories: 481 | Fat: 18.1 g | Protein: 30.0 g | Sodium: 222 mg | Fiber: 7.6 g | Carbohydrates: 47.7 g | Sugar: 30.5 g

Chickpeas or Garbanzo Beans?

Chickpeas and garbanzo beans aren't two different things; they're one and the same! The English word "chickpea" comes from the French word *pois chiche*. *Garbanzo* is the name in Spanish. Both can be used interchangeably, depending upon personal preference. Chickpeas have been cultivated for thousands of years and are a staple in many diets around the world. They have a buttery, nutlike flavor that pairs wonderfully with many foods, both sweet and savory. They are high in protein and fiber, very low in fat, and are a rich source of many important vitamins and minerals.

Vegan Mac 'n' Cheese

This tried-and-true recipe is a delicious favorite. Addictively gooey and filled with cheesy flavor—without any actual cheese!—it's the best vegan mac and cheese you'll ever make! This MIND diet dish is delicious, inexpensive, and table-ready in just 25 minutes.

PREP TIME: 5 minutes
COOK TIME: 20 minutes

INGREDIENTS | SERVES 8

1 (16-ounce) package whole-grain pasta shells
3 tablespoons olive oil
2 tablespoons white whole-wheat flour
2 tablespoons nutritional yeast
1 teaspoon all-purpose seasoning
¼ teaspoon freshly ground black pepper
1 cup vegetable broth
1 cup shredded vegan (soy-free) cheese

1. Cook pasta according to package directions. Drain and set aside.

2. Place a medium saucepan over medium heat and add oil, flour, nutritional yeast, seasoning, and pepper. Whisk well to combine. The mixture will be thick and paste-like.

3. Add broth and whisk well to combine. Cook, stirring constantly, until mixture is thick and bubbly, roughly 3–5 minutes.

4. Add cheese and stir until smooth.

5. Remove from heat, pour cheese sauce over pasta, and stir until combined.

6. Serve immediately.

PER SERVING Calories: 312 | Fat: 9.3 g | Protein: 10.0 g | Sodium: 153 mg | Fiber: 6.5 g | Carbohydrates: 47.2 g | Sugar: 1.3 g

Potato Latkes

These delicious potato pancakes are a perfect accompaniment to breakfast, lunch, or dinner, but are filling enough to eat on their own. Season them as desired; try them plain or topped with applesauce, ketchup, or even sour cream. Whether you like them sweet or savory—or just the way they are—you'll find yourself making them again and again.

PREP TIME: 10 minutes
COOK TIME: 18–30 minutes

INGREDIENTS | SERVES 6

6 medium potatoes, peeled and grated

1 small onion, peeled and grated

2 large eggs, beaten

2 tablespoons unbleached all-purpose flour

1 tablespoon white whole-wheat flour

½ teaspoon freshly ground black pepper

¼ teaspoon ground nutmeg

1 cup olive oil

1. Place potato and onion in a large mixing bowl. Add eggs, flours, pepper, and nutmeg and stir well to combine.

2. Heat oil in a large skillet over medium-high heat. Add ⅓ cup potato mixture to hot oil, flatten slightly with a spatula, and cook until golden brown and crisp on bottom, about 3–5 minutes. Flip gently and brown on second side another 3–5 minutes.

3. Remove from pan and drain on paper towels. Repeat process with remaining potato mixture.

4. Serve warm.

PER SERVING Calories: 262 | Fat: 13.3 g | Protein: 5.0 g | Sodium: 346 mg | Fiber: 3.2 g | Carbohydrates: 30.9 g | Sugar: 1.7 g

Potato Facts

Did you know that potatoes are a fantastic source of vitamin C? It's true! One medium potato (with the skin left on) contains 45 percent of the daily recommended value of vitamin C, more than half a grapefruit! They're also high in vitamin B_6, iron, magnesium, fiber, and protein. Native to South America, potatoes are now grown worldwide and have become one of the biggest agricultural crops of Europe, China, and India.

Garlic Knots

The texture of these delicious Garlic Knots is pure comfort. Each pillowy mound is so soft and tender, you'll want to rest your head on its folds and go to sleep. Good thing there's no kneading required and very little cleanup!

PREP TIME: 4 hours
COOK TIME: 15 minutes

INGREDIENTS | YIELDS 3 DOZEN

1¾ cups lukewarm water

6 tablespoons olive oil, divided

1 tablespoon sugar

1½ tablespoons dry active yeast

5 cups unbleached all-purpose flour

½ cup white whole-wheat flour

2 tablespoons unsalted butter

4 cloves garlic, finely minced

¼ cup finely chopped fresh flat-leaf parsley

1. To make the dough, add water, 4 tablespoons olive oil, sugar, and yeast in a large mixing bowl and whisk well to combine. Whisk flours together in a clean medium mixing bowl. Add to yeast mixture ½ cup at a time and stir well to combine. Cover the bowl with plastic wrap and set someplace warm to rise. Let rise until doubled in size, roughly 1–3 hours.

2. Cover two baking sheets with parchment; set aside.

3. Turn dough out onto a lightly floured surface. Lightly oil your hands to keep dough from sticking to them. Divide dough into two equal parts for ease; set one half aside. Roll dough out into a 16" × 5" rectangle using a lightly oiled rolling pin. Slice dough into 18 (½") strips using a pizza cutter.

4. Gently roll each strip into a short rope, then tie the rope into a little knot. Note: sprinkle dough liberally with flour to prevent dough from sticking and make knot tying simple. Place the tied knots on the baking sheet 2" apart.

5. Repeat process with the remaining half of the dough, then place sheets in a warm place to rise until doubled in size, roughly 30 minutes.

continued on next page

6. Preheat oven to 400°F. Once knots have doubled in size, place baking sheets on middle rack in oven. Bake 7–8 minutes, switch sheet positions (to ensure even browning), and bake an additional 7–8 minutes or until golden.

7. While knots are baking, gently warm remaining 2 tablespoons oil, butter, and garlic in a small saucepan until butter has melted and garlic has softened. Remove from heat, add parsley, and stir to combine. Set aside.

8. Remove knots from oven and brush with garlic coating or place knots in a large bowl and toss with garlic coating. Serve immediately.

PER KNOT Calories: 97 | Fat: 3.0 g | Protein: 2.3 g | Sodium: 1 mg | Fiber: 0.9 g | Carbohydrates: 15.2 g | Sugar: 0.4 g

French Onion Soup

A healthier take on the classic, this French Onion Soup is made with a real French baguette and Swiss cheese and is perfect for those times when you decide to add cheese and butter to your diet. Go ahead and savor each melty, heavenly bite.

PREP TIME: 15 minutes
COOK TIME: 1 hour 40 minutes

INGREDIENTS | SERVES 8

2 tablespoons plus 1 teaspoon olive oil
2 tablespoons unsalted butter
4 large onions, peeled and thinly sliced
½ teaspoon freshly ground black pepper
1 teaspoon sugar
1 small French baguette, cut into ½" slices
8 cups beef broth
1 bay leaf
8 slices Swiss cheese

1. Heat 2 tablespoons oil and butter in a medium stockpot over medium heat until butter has melted. Stir in onions and pepper. Reduce heat to low.

2. Press a piece of foil onto onions to cover completely, cover the pot with a lid, and cook stirring occasionally until onions are very soft but not falling apart, 40–50 minutes.

3. Remove the lid and foil, raise the heat to medium-high, and stir in sugar. Cook stirring often until onions are very deeply browned, 10–15 minutes.

4. To make baguette toasts, preheat oven to 350°F. Lightly oil a rimmed baking sheet with remaining oil and arrange slices on the sheet in a single layer. Place sheet on the middle rack in oven and bake 7–10 minutes; turn bread and bake 7–10 minutes until bread is crisp and lightly browned. Remove from oven and set aside.

5. Add broth and bay leaf to onions and bring to a boil over medium-high heat. Reduce the heat to medium-low and simmer 10 minutes. Discard bay leaf.

6. To serve, position oven rack 6" from the broiler and heat the broiler to high. Place 8 ovenproof soup bowls on a baking sheet. Arrange bread slices in the bottom of each bowl and ladle the hot soup on top. Top each bowl with a slice of cheese. Place soup under broiler and broil until the tops are browned and bubbly, 2–5 minutes.

7. Remove from oven and serve immediately.

PER SERVING Calories: 299 | Fat: 15.0 g | Protein: 14.6 g | Sodium: 1,106 mg | Fiber: 1.9 g | Carbohydrates: 25.0 g | Sugar: 5.2 g

Tuscan Lemon Muffins

Let these muffins transport your taste buds to Tuscany. These muffins are light and airy thanks to the ricotta cheese, and are flecked with grated lemon zest with a crunch of raw sugar on top. Each moist, subtly sweet bite is a feast for the senses, heightened by the flavor of olive oil.

PREP TIME: 10 minutes
COOK TIME: 16 minutes

INGREDIENTS | YIELDS 1 DOZEN

1½ cups unbleached all-purpose flour
¼ cup white whole-wheat flour
¾ cup sugar
2½ teaspoons baking powder
¾ cup low-fat ricotta cheese
½ cup water
¼ cup olive oil
1 large egg
Juice and grated zest of
1 medium lemon
Olive oil cooking spray
2 tablespoons demerara (coarse) sugar

1. Preheat oven to 375°F. Line a 12-muffin tin with paper liners and set aside.

2. Measure flours, sugar, and baking powder into a large mixing bowl and whisk well to combine. In a medium mixing bowl, combine ricotta, water, oil, egg, and lemon zest and juice; whisk well. Add ricotta mixture to flour mixture and stir until just moist.

3. Spray muffin cups lightly with olive oil spray, then divide batter evenly among muffin cups. Sprinkle ½ teaspoon coarse sugar over each muffin.

4. Place pan on middle rack in oven and bake 16 minutes until lightly golden.

5. Remove pan from oven and place on a wire rack to cool 5 minutes.

6. Remove muffins from tin and serve immediately.

PER MUFFIN Calories: 191 | Fat: 6.0 g | Protein: 4.3 g | Sodium: 123 mg | Fiber: 0.8 g | Carbohydrates: 30.2 g | Sugar: 15.2 g

Different Types of Sugar

Cane sugar comes in many different varieties, the three standard types being white granulated sugar, brown sugar, and powdered or confectioners' sugar. But there are other alternatives. Evaporated cane sugar, also called raw or turbinado sugar, is a natural, unrefined product that can be substituted one for one for granulated sugar. Demerara sugar is similar to raw sugar, but with a larger, coarser grain. It's often sprinkled on muffins or scones before baking.

Chocolate-Drizzled Almond Biscotti

Don't waste your money on overpriced coffeehouse biscotti. Those aren't great when you're following the MIND diet and when it's so easy to make your own! These delicious Italian cookies have a double dose of almond: extract in the batter and slivered nuts on top. If you own an electric mixer, use it when making this batter; it'll save your arm a good workout.

PREP TIME: 20 minutes
COOK TIME: 35 minutes

INGREDIENTS | YIELDS 2½ DOZEN

½ cup plus 2 teaspoons olive oil, divided
1 cup sugar
1 tablespoon vanilla extract
1½ teaspoons almond extract
3 large eggs
1 tablespoon baking powder
3½ cups unbleached all-purpose flour
½ cup semisweet chocolate chips
¼ cup chopped or slivered almonds

1. Preheat oven to 375°F. Lightly grease two baking sheets with 1 teaspoon olive oil and set aside.

2. In a large mixing bowl, beat sugar with ½ cup oil, vanilla, and almond extract. Add eggs one at a time and beat well after each addition. Stir in baking powder. Gradually add in flour and mix well; scrape the sides of the bowl to incorporate.

3. Lightly flour your hands, then divide the dough into two equal parts. The dough may be sticky—this is normal. Just lightly reflour your hands as necessary.

4. Roll each of the two dough parts into a roughly 8"-long cylinder. Place cylinders onto individual baking sheets, then lightly press each cylinder down to flatten to about 1½" thickness.

5. Place baking sheets on the middle rack in the oven and bake 25 minutes.

6. Remove sheets from oven, let rest 1 minute, then carefully slice the baked loaves with a serrated knife into 1" slices.

7. Gently place the cookies cut-side down onto the baking sheets. Place sheets on middle rack in oven and bake 5 minutes. Gently flip cookies over and bake 3 minutes until lightly toasted. Remove from oven and carefully transfer cookies to a wire rack.

continued on next page

Chocolate-Drizzled Almond Biscotti–continued

8. Place chocolate chips and the remaining teaspoon olive oil in a microwave-safe bowl or mug. Microwave 40 seconds on high. Remove from microwave and stir until smooth. Heat another 10 seconds if chips have not melted fully.

9. Drizzle chocolate over cookies and immediately sprinkle with almonds.

10. Let cookies rest until chocolate has completely hardened, then store in an airtight container for up to 5 days. To speed up hardening of chocolate, place cookies in the refrigerator or freezer 10 minutes.

PER BISCOTTI Calories: 131 | Fat: 4.9 | Protein: 2.4 g | Sodium: 56 mg | Fiber: 0.6 g | Carbohydrates: 18.9 g | Sugar: 7.4 g

Foolproof Fabulous Brownies

*This dish gives you rich, dense, and supremely chocolatey brownies—
in an easy, foolproof recipe! Dutch-processed cocoa produces a
much deeper, more complex flavor, but standard cocoa works just
fine, too. Add ¼ cup chopped nuts to the batter if desired.*

PREP TIME: 10 minutes
COOK TIME: 30 minutes

INGREDIENTS | YIELDS 2 DOZEN

⅓ cup plus 1 teaspoon olive oil, divided

¾ cup plus 1 tablespoon unbleached
all-purpose flour, divided

3 large eggs

1½ cups sugar

1 teaspoon vanilla extract

1 cup unsweetened cocoa powder

½ cup unsalted butter, melted

1 cup semisweet chocolate chips

What Is Cocoa Powder?

Cocoa powder comes from the leftover sol-
ids that remain after cocoa butter is
extracted from cacao beans. These crum-
bly residual bits are ground into a fine powder, making cocoa. The essence of
chocolate, without any added fat or sweetness, cocoa can be used in a myriad of
ways. Standard cocoa powder is slightly
acidic, with a pH between 5 and 6. Dutch-
processed cocoa is washed with a solution
of potassium carbonate that changes its
acidity, leaving it with a neutral pH of 7 or
slightly alkaline pH of 8. The process
changes the cocoa, giving it a darker
brown color and more intense chocolate flavor.

1. Preheat oven to 350°F. Grease and flour the bottom and sides of a 9" × 13" pan with 1 teaspoon olive oil and 1 tablespoon flour; set aside.

2. In a medium bowl, beat together eggs, sugar, and vanilla. Add cocoa, butter, and oil and mix well. Stir in flour, then add chocolate chips. Scrape the bottom of the bowl to make sure everything is well incorporated.

3. Spread the thick batter into the prepared pan and smooth top to even. Place on middle rack in oven and bake exactly 30 minutes; do not bake any longer! Even if the brownies appear a little loose in the center, they will firm up fully after cooling.

4. Remove pan from oven and place on a wire rack to cool completely. Cut into slices and serve only after the brownies have completely cooled.

PER BROWNIE Calories: 153 | Fat: 8.2 g | Protein: 2.1 g | Sodium: 12 mg | Fiber: 1.6 g | Carbohydrates: 19.3 g | Sugar: 14.1 g

Pumpkin Whoopie Pies

Spicy, moist, and irresistible, these whoopie pies are packed with vitamin-rich pumpkin and a sweet cream-cheese filling. A few notes about the recipe. 1) Yes! You really do use that much spice, so don't skimp. 2) Save yourself hassle or heartache and line your baking sheets with parchment. 3) Make sure you've eaten before making these; otherwise, you'll find yourself going overboard. Enjoy!

PREP TIME: 45 minutes
COOK TIME: 15 minutes

INGREDIENTS | YIELDS 1 DOZEN

2½ cups unbleached all-purpose flour
½ cup white whole-wheat flour
2 teaspoons baking powder
1 teaspoon baking soda
2 tablespoons ground cinnamon
1 tablespoon ground ginger
1 tablespoon ground cloves
2 cups packed brown sugar
1 cup olive oil
3 cups chilled pumpkin purée
2 large eggs
2 teaspoons vanilla extract, divided
3 cups powdered sugar
4 tablespoons unsalted butter, softened
2 ounces cream cheese, softened
4 tablespoons low-fat milk

1. Preheat oven to 350°F. Line two baking sheets with parchment and set aside.

2. In a large bowl, whisk together flours, baking powder, baking soda, cinnamon, ginger, and cloves; set aside.

3. In another large bowl, mix together brown sugar and oil. Add pumpkin and stir until combined. Add eggs and 1 teaspoon vanilla and mix until well combined. Gradually add flour mixture and stir until fully incorporated.

4. Use a small retractable ice-cream scoop and drop heaping tablespoons of dough onto the prepared baking sheets about 1" apart. Transfer to oven and bake on middle rack 15 minutes, until set. Remove from oven and let cool completely on pan, roughly 30 minutes.

5. To make the filling, sift powdered sugar into a small mixing bowl. Add butter and cream cheese and beat until smooth. Add milk and remaining 1 teaspoon vanilla and beat until fluffy.

6. When cookies have cooled completely, pipe or spread a large dollop of filling on the flat side of one of the cookies. Sandwich with another cookie and press down slightly so that the filling spreads to the edges. Transfer to a plate or cover with plastic wrap. Repeat with remaining cookies and filling. Serve immediately or cover cookies with plastic wrap and refrigerate up to 3 days.

PER WHOOPIE PIE Calories: 589 | Fat: 23.7 g | Protein: 5.6 g | Sodium: 232 mg | Fiber: 3.6 g | Carbohydrates: 89.4 g | Sugar: 61.7 g

Resources

Alzheimer's Association

225 N. Michigan Avenue, Floor 17
Chicago, IL 60601
800-272-3900

www.alz.org

The Alzheimer's Association is the leading voluntary health organization in Alzheimer's care, support, and research.

Alzheimer's Foundation of America (AFA)

322 Eighth Avenue, 7th Floor
New York, NY 10001
866-232-8484

www.alzfdn.org

The Alzheimer's Foundation of America (AFA) was founded by a consortium of organizations to fill the gap that existed on a national level to assure quality of care and excellence in service to individuals with Alzheimer's disease and related illnesses, and to their caregivers and families.

California Gold Dust

290 West Main Street
Northboro, MA 01532
508-393-7625

www.californiagolddust.com

California Gold Dust is a turmeric supplement product that contains black pepper, which contains a compound that boosts the absorption rate of curcumin by 2,000 percent.

Gaia Herbs

101 Gaia Herbs Drive
Brevard, NC 28712
800-831-7780

www.gaiaherbs.com

Gaia Herbs offers pure, potent herbal supplements, including ginkgo, that can help boost brain power, increase mental clarity, and improve focus.

Mayo Clinic: Calorie Calculator

www.mayoclinic.org/healthy-lifestyle/nutrition-and-healthy-eating/in-depth/calorie-calculator/itt-20084939

The Mayo Clinic Calorie Calculator can be used to determine how many calories you need to take in each day based on your age, height, weight, and activity. To adjust calories for weight loss, subtract 500 calories from calculated amount.

U.S. News & World Report

http://health.usnews.com/best-diet/mind-diet

See how the MIND diet rates compared to other popular diets of 2016.

MIND Diet Food Lists

Whole Grains

Amaranth

Barley

Buckwheat

Millet

Oats

Quinoa

Rice (brown and wild)

Rye

Sorghum

Teff

Triticale

Wheat

Green Leafy Vegetables

Arugula

Chicory

Collard greens

Dandelion greens

Kale

Leaf lettuce

Mustard greens

Romaine lettuce

Spinach

Swiss chard

Other Vegetables

Acorn squash

Artichoke

Asparagus

Bell peppers (all color varieties)

Beets

Bok Choy

Broccoli

Brussels sprouts

Butternut squash

Carrots

Cauliflower

Celery

Cucumbers

Eggplant

Green beans

Mushrooms

Onions

Radish

Snap peas

Spaghetti squash

Sweet potatoes

Tomatoes

Turnips

Zucchini

Fruit

All fruits are allowed, but blueberries are the only fruit specifically recommended

Blueberries

Beans and Legumes

Black beans

Black-eyed peas

Fava beans

Garbanzo beans (chickpeas)

Kidney beans

Lentils

Navy beans

Pinto beans

White beans

Fats and Oils

Avocado

Avocado oil

Coconut

Flaxseed oil

Olive oil (olive oil is the recommended cooking and eating oil, but other oils are also allowed)

Olives

Nuts and Seeds

Almond butter

Almonds

Cashew butter

Cashews

Pistachios

Pumpkin seeds

Sesame seeds

Sunflower seed butter

Sunflower seeds

Walnuts

Spices, Herbs, and Other Allowed Foods

All herbs and spices are allowed, but these are especially beneficial for brain health

Balsamic vinegar

Basil

Cinnamon

Curcumin (turmeric)

Curry

Garlic

Ginger

Low-fat plain yogurt

Marjoram

Mustard

Oregano

Rosemary

Saffron

Sage

Thyme

Standard Metric/U.S. Measurement Conversion Chart

VOLUME CONVERSIONS

U.S. Volume Measure	Metric Equivalent
⅛ teaspoon	0.5 milliliter
¼ teaspoon	1 milliliter
½ teaspoon	2 milliliters
1 teaspoon	5 milliliters
½ tablespoon	7 milliliters
1 tablespoon (3 teaspoons)	15 milliliters
2 tablespoons (1 fluid ounce)	30 milliliters
¼ cup (4 tablespoons)	60 milliliters
⅓ cup	90 milliliters
½ cup (4 fluid ounces)	125 milliliters
⅔ cup	160 milliliters
¾ cup (6 fluid ounces)	180 milliliters
1 cup (16 tablespoons)	250 milliliters
1 pint (2 cups)	500 milliliters
1 quart (4 cups)	1 liter (about)

WEIGHT CONVERSIONS

U.S. Weight Measure	Metric Equivalent
½ ounce	15 grams
1 ounce	30 grams
2 ounces	60 grams
3 ounces	85 grams
¼ pound (4 ounces)	115 grams
½ pound (8 ounces)	225 grams
¾ pound (12 ounces)	340 grams
1 pound (16 ounces)	454 grams

OVEN TEMPERATURE CONVERSIONS

Degrees Fahrenheit	Degrees Celsius
200 degrees F	95 degrees C
250 degrees F	120 degrees C
275 degrees F	135 degrees C
300 degrees F	150 degrees C
325 degrees F	160 degrees C
350 degrees F	180 degrees C
375 degrees F	190 degrees C
400 degrees F	205 degrees C
425 degrees F	220 degrees C
450 degrees F	230 degrees C

BAKING PAN SIZES

American	Metric
8 x 1½ inch round baking pan	20 x 4 cm cake tin
9 x 1½ inch round baking pan	23 x 3.5 cm cake tin
11 x 7 x 1½ inch baking pan	28 x 18 x 4 cm baking tin
13 x 9 x 2 inch baking pan	30 x 20 x 5 cm baking tin
2 quart rectangular baking dish	30 x 20 x 3 cm baking tin
15 x 10 x 2 inch baking pan	30 x 25 x 2 cm baking tin (Swiss roll tin)
9 inch pie plate	22 x 4 or 23 x 4 cm pie plate
7 or 8 inch springform pan	18 or 20 cm springform or loose bottom cake tin
9 x 5 x 3 inch loaf pan	23 x 13 x 7 cm or 2 lb narrow loaf or pate tin
1½ quart casserole	1.5 liter casserole
2 quart casserole	2 liter casserole

Index